Transformational Leadership

Renewing Fundamental Values and Achieving
New Relationships in Health Care

MARY K. KOHLES, RN, MSW
WILLIAM G. BAKER, JR., MD
BARBARA A. DONAHO, RN, MA

AHA books are published by American Hospital Publishing, Inc., an American Hospital Association company

This publication is designed to provide accurate and authoritative information in regard to the subject matter covered. It is sold with the understanding that neither the author nor the publisher is engaged in rendering legal, accounting, or other professional service. If legal advice or other expert assistance is required, the services of a competent professional should be sought.

The views expressed in this book are solely those of the authors and contributors; official endorsement by the Robert Wood Johnson Foundation, the Pew Charitable Trusts, or the American Hospital Association is not intended and should not be inferred.

Library of Congress Cataloging-in-Publication Data

Kohles, Mary K.
  Transformational leadership : renewing fundamental values and
achieving new relationships in health care / Mary K. Kohles, William
G. Baker, Jr., and Barbara A. Donaho.
      p.   cm.
  Includes bibliographical references.
  ISBN 1-55648-144-6
  1. Health services administration.   2. Leadership.
3. Organizational change.   I. Baker, William G., 1936–
II. Donaho, Barbara A.   III. Title.
  [DNLM: 1. Hospital Administration.   2. Leadership.
3. Organizational Innovation.   WX 150 K793t 1995]
RA971.K58   1995
362.1'068'4 — dc20
DNLM/DLC
for Library of Congress   95-35494
                                                                           CIP

Catalog no. 001116

All rights reserved. The reproduction or use of this book in any form or in any information storage or retrieval system is forbidden without the express written permission of the publisher.

Printed in the USA

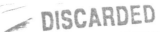

Text set in English Times
3M—10/95—0424
3M—08/96—0447
Cover illustration by Mary Flock Lempa

Linda Conheady, Senior Editor
Nancy Charpentier, Editor
Peggy DuMais, Production Coordinator
Luke Smith, Cover Designer
Marcia Bottoms, Executive Editor
Brian Schenk, Books Division Director

Dedicated in memory of Brian Schenk,
whose leadership and vision were an inspiration
to all who knew him

Contents

List of Figures and Tables

About the Authors

Mary K. Kohles, RN, MSW, is the deputy director of the national program, Strengthening Hospital Nursing: A Program to Improve Patient Care (SHNP). The SHNP grant is cosponsored by the Robert Wood Johnson Foundation and the Pew Charitable Trusts with direction and technical assistance provided by Children's Research Institute, Inc., All Children's Hospital, St. Petersburg, Florida. Ms. Kohles is also the deputy director for the national program, Ladders in Nursing Careers (LINC) funded by the Robert Wood Johnson Foundation with direction and technical assistance provided by the Greater New York Hospital Foundation, Inc., New York City.

Before joining the grant in 1988, Ms. Kohles held administrative positions, nursing and operations, at Bellin Hospital, Green Bay, Wisconsin, and University of Wisconsin Hospital and Clinics, Madison. She has held critical care staff and management positions in community, university, and military settings.

Ms. Kohles has experience in health care planning and policy at community and state levels. She has presented and published information related to SHNP, including organizational culture transitions, work and role design, continuity of care delivery systems, and linkages that promote integration of the health care system with the community and educational institutions. She has served as a volunteer for community development projects relating to building a healthier community status in St. Petersburg, Florida.

Ms. Kohles received a BSN from Mount Marty College, Yankton, South Dakota, and an MSW from the University of Nebraska, Lincoln.

William G. Baker, Jr., MD, is vice-president of medical services at Piedmont Hospital (a member of the Promina Health System) in Atlanta. He is also an associate with Hunter Group, a health care consulting firm in St. Petersburg, Florida. Previously he was medical director at St. Anthony's Hospital in St. Petersburg, Florida.

Dr. Baker moved to St. Petersburg in 1968 to join the St. Petersburg Medical Clinic, where he practiced consulting gastroenterology for 25 years, with clinical privileges at all the major hospitals in St. Petersburg. During this time, he served as president of the St. Petersburg Medical Clinic and as chief of staff and governing board member of St. Anthony's Hospital. He was also a clinical associate professor of Medicine at the University of South Florida.

Dr. Baker has presented and published numerous articles in his medical specialty. His recent presentations and publications are in the areas of quality (value) improvement, organizational development, organizational soul, and the leadership role for physicians in health care systems. He has served as president of the Florida Gastroenterological Association and was founding president of the Florida Society for Gastrointestinal Endoscopy. He was active in the St. Petersburg community, serving as president of the St. Petersburg High School PTSA, St. Thomas Church warden, and president of the St. Petersburg Free Clinic.

Dr. Baker graduated from Emory University School of Medicine as a member of Phi Beta Kappa and Alpha Omega Alpha, the honorary medical society. He received his specialty training at the Massachusetts General Hospital and the New York Hospital Cornell Medical Center.

Barbara A. Donaho, RN, MA, FAAN, is the director of the national program, Strengthening Hospital Nursing: A Program to Improve Patient Care (SHNP). The SHNP grant is cosponsored by the Robert Wood Johnson Foundation and the Pew Charitable Trusts with direction and technical assistance provided by Children's Research Institute, Inc., All Children's Hospital, St. Petersburg, Florida. She previously was president/CEO of St. Anthony's Hospital and Health Care Center in St. Petersburg, Florida.

Before joining St. Anthony's, Ms. Donaho was the vice-president for nursing and patient care at Shands Hospital at the University of Florida, Gainesville. She held corporate-level positions at Sisters of Mercy Health Corporation, Farmington Hills, Michigan, and executive level positions at Hartford Hospital, Hartford, Connecticut, and Abbott-Northwestern Hospital, Minneapolis. She had the honor of being the first nurse member of the American Hospital Association board of directors. Ms. Donaho has served as a commissioner of the Joint Commission on Accreditation of Health Care Organizations (JCAHO) representing the American Hospital Association, and she chaired the American Hospital Association's Council on Nursing. She was a member of the board of governors, Cathedral Healthcare System, Newark, New Jersey, and a member of the board of trustees, Catherine McAuley Health System, Ann Arbor, Michigan. She is currently a trustee for Johns Hopkins University, Baltimore, and the Sisters of Providence Health System, Seattle, Washington. She received the distinguished alumnus of the year award from Johns Hopkins University, the trustee award from the American Hospital Association, and the 1992 quality award from the Society for Healthcare Planning and Marketing, Santa Barbara, California.

Ms. Donaho holds a BSN degree from Johns Hopkins University and an MA from the University of Chicago. She has held faculty appointments at the University of Michigan, the University of Minnesota, and Boston University. She is a member and past president of the American Organization of Nurse Executives, and will assume the presidency of the American Academy of Nurses in the fall of 1995. She is a member of the fellows of the American Academy of Nurses and Johnson & Johnson-Wharton Fellows Program. She has presented and published information relating to SHNP and lectured extensively on management and organizational change with a continuing focus on multidisciplinary patient care delivery systems.

Contributors

Sharon Aadalen, RN, PhD, consortium director, Health BOND, and associate professor, School of Nursing, Mankato State University, Mankato, Minnesota

Rhonda Anderson, RN, MPA, CNAA, vice-president, patient operations, Hartford Hospital, Hartford, Connecticut

Marianne D. Araujo, RN, MSN, senior manager, Ernst and Young Midwest, Park Ridge, Illinois

Arlene Austinson, RN, MN, assistant administrator, nursing and patient care services, Providence Portland Medical Center, Portland, Oregon

Wendy L. Baker, RN, MS, staff associate, Office of the Senior Associate Director, University of Michigan Hospital, Ann Arbor, Michigan

Alan M. Barstow, PhD, Barstow & Associates, Philadelphia

Susan Beck, RN, PhD, project director, University Hospital's Program to Improve Patient Care, and nurse researcher, University Hospital/University of Utah, Salt Lake City

Chris Beebe, member, board of trustees, Northeast Health Consortium, Rockport, Maine

George W. Belsey, MBA, chairman/CEO, Air Methods Corporation, Denver International Airport, Englewood, Colorado (former executive director, University Hospital/University of Utah, Salt Lake City)

Marjorie Beyers, RN, PhD, FAAN, SHNP National Advisory Committee member; co-project director, SHNP project, Mercy Health Services, Farmington

Hills, Michigan; and executive director, American Organization of Nurse Executives, Chicago

Brad Brown, vice-president, management information systems, Tallahassee Memorial Regional Medical Center, Tallahassee, Florida

Colleen Burch, RN, assistant head nurse, neurology, urology, ENT, gynecology, and pediatric unit, Providence Portland Medical Center, Portland, Oregon

Mark A. Burzynski, president/CEO, Yellowstone Community Health Plan, Billings, Montana (former CFO, Saint Vincent Hospital and Health Center, Billings, and the SHNP project, Montana Consortium for Excellence in Health Care, Billings)

Joe Caroselli, CEO, Idaho Elk's Rehabilitation Hospital, Boise, Idaho

Martin P. Charns, DBA, SHNP National Advisory Committee member and director, Management Decision & Research Center, Health Services Research and Development Service, Department of Veterans Affairs, Boston

Mark Chastang, president/CEO, East Orange General Hospital, East Orange, New Jersey (former executive director, District of Columbia Hospital, Washington, DC)

Joyce C. Clifford, RN, MSN, FAAN, SHNP National Advisory Committee member and vice-president, nursing, and nurse-in-chief, Beth Israel Hospital, Boston

Annette Compton, director of volunteers, St. Luke's Regional Medical Center, Boise, Idaho

Pamela Copeland, JD, risk manager and acting director for legal risk services, District of Columbia General Hospital, Washington, DC

Edward E. Dahlberg, president, St. Luke's Regional Medical Center, Boise, Idaho

Paula Delahanty, RN, director, quality management department, Penobscot Bay Medical Center, Rockport, Maine (former project director, Integrated Care System, Northeast Health Consortium, Rockport, Maine)

Joan M. Lartin-Drake, RN, PhD, project director, Horizons — Partnership in Patient Care, University Hospitals/Pennsylvania State University at The Milton S. Hershey Medical Center, Hershey, Pennsylvania

Marie J. Driever, RN, PhD, co-project director, redesign and improvement for patient care delivery, and assistant director, nursing for quality research, Providence Portland Medical Center, Portland, Oregon

Laura J. Duprat, RN, MS, MPH, project director, integrated clinical practice, Beth Israel Hospital, Boston, Massachusetts

Shirley Edwards, RN, acting associate administrator, nursing, District of Columbia General Hospital, Washington, DC

Stephen S. Entman, MD, professor/vice-chair, obstetrics and gynecology, Vanderbilt University Hospital, Nashville

Geraldene Felton, RN, EdD, FAAN, SHNP National Advisory Committee member and professor/dean, College of Nursing, University of Iowa, Iowa City, Iowa

Dominick L. Flarey, PhD, MBA, RN, CCNAA, administrator/COO, Youngstown Osteopathic Hospital, Youngstown, Ohio; and executive consultant, Coopers & Lybrand Consulting, Chicago and Niles, Ohio

Linda Fleury, human resource analyst, MeritCare Health System, Fargo, North Dakota

Edward J. Foley, regional vice-president, Hospital Council of Southern California, Center of Health Resources, Santa Ana, California

Wayne R. Frieders, vice-president, human resources, St. Luke's Regional Medical Center, Boise, Idaho

Susan R. Goldsmith, MS, project coordinator, Community of Patient Care Leaders, Harbor-UCLA Medical Center, Torrance, California

Winifred M. Hageman, SHNP National Advisory Committee member and principal, The Umbdenstock-Hageman Partnership, Seattle

Ruth B. Hanson, RN, MA, project director, Reaching In, Reaching Out, and Reaching Beyond, MeritCare Hospital, Fargo, North Dakota

Evelyn G. Hartigan, RN, EdD, associate administrator, patient care services, University Hospital/University of Utah, Salt Lake City

Al Herzog, MD, vice-president, medical affairs, Hartford Hospital, Hartford, Connecticut

Nancy J. Higgerson, RN, MA, SHNP National Advisory Committee member and vice-president, nursing, the Moses H. Cone Memorial Hospital, Greensboro, North Carolina

Peggy W. Hughes, JD, secretary, board of directors, Tallahassee Memorial Regional Medical Center, Tallahassee, Florida

Barbara Hunt, RN, nurse manager, pediatric emergency room and pediatric outpatient department, District of Columbia General Hospital, Washington, DC

Carolyn T. Hunt, RN, MS, associate vice-president, patient care services, Liberty Medical Center, Baltimore

Gloria Jacks, RN, assistant director, Unit Two West, National Rehabilitation Hospital, Washington, DC

Howard Jessamy, chair, advisory committee for the Patient-Centered Care Delivery System, District of Columbia Hospital Association, Washington, DC

Lawrence T. Johnson, MD, medical director, District of Columbia General Hospital, Washington, DC

Maryalice Jordan-Marsh, RN, PhD, director, nursing research, Community of Patient Care Leaders, Harbor-UCLA Medical Center, Torrance, California

Toni H. Kaeding, RN, MSA, project director, Vermont Nursing Initiative, Montpelier, Vermont

Fran Kauffman, RN, nurse manager, orthopedic/urology unit, District of Columbia General Hospital, Washington, DC

Alan Kinne, administrator, Knox Center for Long-Term Care, a division of Penobscot Bay Medical Center; and member, steering committee, Integrated Care System, Northeast Health Consortium, Rockport, Maine

Cheryl Kinnear, RN, BSN, project manager, University Hospital's Program to Improve Patient Care, University Hospital/University of Utah, Salt Lake City

John F. Lathrop, PhD, director, Strategic Insights, Los Altos, California

Sharon A. Lee, RN, MBA, vice-president, patient care services, St. Luke's Regional Medical Center, Boise, Idaho

Richard W. Lindsay, MD, SHNP National Advisory Committee member and professor of medicine, and head, Division of Geriatric Medicine, School of Medicine, University of Virginia, Charlottesville, Virginia

Elaine A. LoGuidice, RN, MSN, CNAA, project director, Patient-Centered Care Delivery System, District of Columbia General Hospital, Washington, DC

Richard Lopez, MD, director, substance abuse program, District of Columbia Hospital, Washington, DC

Ginger Malone, RN, MSN, project director, "INNOVATION—The Nature of Change," and nurse leader and consultant, community care and case management, Abbott-Northwestern Hospital, Minneapolis

William D. Manahan, MD, medical director, quality assurance, Immanuel-St. Joseph's Hospital, Mankato, Minnesota

Michael Marby, administrative sergeant, hospital police, District of Columbia Hospital, Washington, DC

Lynne Meredith Mattison, MHA, consortium project director, the Montana Consortium for Excellence in Health Care, Billings, Montana

Annette J. McBeth, RN, MS, vice-president, Immanuel-St. Joseph's Hospital, Mankato, Minnesota

John Meehan, president/CEO, Hartford Hospital, Hartford, Connecticut

Cassandra Morgan, RN, director, medical nursing, and acting director, nursing education, District of Columbia General Hospital, Washington, DC

Thomas C. Mroczkowski, vice-president/COO, Hackley Hospital, Muskegon, Michigan

Ann Murchland, RN, clinical specialist, department of maternal child health, District of Columbia General Hospital, Washington, DC

Connie Murphy, project coordinator, patient driven care project, Mercy Hospital and Medical Center, Chicago

Peggy J. Nazarey, RN, MSN, director, nursing, and project director, Community of Patient Care Leaders, Harbor-UCLA Medical Center, Torrance, California

Susan Neves, LMSW, geriatric facilitator, Northeast Health Integrated Care System, Northeast Health Consortium, Rockport, Maine

Anne Payne, RN, EdD, associate dean/chair, department of nursing, Boise State University, Boise, Idaho

Nikki Polis, RN, PhD, project director, University Hospitals' SHNP Project, University Hospitals of Cleveland, Cleveland

Hank Primas, associate director, environmental services, District of Columbia General Hospital, Washington, DC

Nellie C. Robinson, RN, MS, assistant executive director, patient care services, Howard University Hospital, Washington, DC (former associate administrator, nursing, District of Columbia General Hospital, Washington, DC)

John A. Romas, MPh, JAR and Associates, Mankato, Minnesota

James E. Sauer, Jr., SHNP National Advisory Committee member and senior vice-president/director, Health Care Division, Alexander & Alexander of California, Inc., Pasadena, California

Betty Sayers, MS, group facilitator, Reaching In, Reaching Out, and Reaching Beyond, MeritCare Health System, Fargo, North Dakota

Debra L. Scammon, PhD, professor, College of Business, University of Utah, Salt Lake City

Winifred H. Schmeling, RN, PhD, FAAN, project director, Program to Improve Patient Care, Tallahassee Memorial Regional Medical Center, Tallahassee, Florida

Brian Schrenk, vice-president, St. Luke's Regional Medical Center, Boise, Idaho

Kathryn Schweer, RN, PhD, dean, academic affairs, Allen College of Nursing, Waterloo, Iowa (former dean of Mankato State University School of Nursing, Mankato, Minnesota)

Paula V. Siler, RN, MS, director, professional practice affairs-nursing, and co-project director, Community of Patient Care Leaders, Harbor-UCLA Medical Center, Torrance, California

Robert I. Siver, vice-president, managed care, All Children's Hospital, St. Petersburg, Florida

Jackie A. Smith, PhD, project manager, University Hospital's Program to Improve Patient Care, University Hospital/University of Utah, Salt Lake City

Joanne Smith, RN, facilitator and case coordinator, medical, surgical, and orthopedic unit, Penobscot Bay Medical Center, Rockport, Maine

Lloyd Smith, executive vice-president, MeritCare Health System, and president/CEO, MeritCare Hospital, Fargo, North Dakota

Rachel Smith, RN, MS, former cochair, Patient-Centered Hospital Environment Subcommittee, and former director, nursing education, District of Columbia General Hospital, Washington, DC

William Sonterre, vice-president, acute care systems, Allina Health System, Minneapolis

Bert Sperry, RN, nurse manager, respiratory and medical units, Providence Portland Medical Center, Portland, Oregon

Judy L. Spinella, RN, MBA, director/COO, Vanderbilt University Hospital, Nashville

Nathan Stark, JD, chair, SHNP National Advisory Committee, and president, National Academy of Social Insurance, Washington, DC

Cheryl B. Stetler, RN, PhD, FAAN, project director/director of clinical practice, Patient-Centered Redesign, Hartford Hospital, Hartford, Connecticut

Joni S. Stright, senior vice-president, McCall Memorial Hospital, McCall, Idaho

Jeanette Ullery, RN, consortium project director, the Rural Connection: Linking for Healthier Communities, St. Luke's Regional Medical Center, Boise, Idaho

Norman B. Urmy, executive director, Vanderbilt University Hospital and the Vanderbilt Clinic, Nashville

Bruce L. Van Cleave, MD, vice-president, professional services, and co-project director, SHNP project, Mercy Health Services, Farmington Hills, Michigan

William Zuber, director, occupational therapy and physical therapy department, Penobscot Bay Medical Center, Rockport, Maine (former facilitator, stroke resource group, Integrated Care System, Northeast Health Consortium, Rockport, Maine)

Preface

Health care professionals have always articulated the goal of quality patient care, but when the financing mechanisms changed, survival became the major influencer in decision making.

Some of the most dramatic changes in health delivery began with the passage of Medicare followed by the diagnosis-related group (DRG) categorization payment structure. The latter legislative action focused attention on costs and resulted in dramatic decreases in length of stay as the initial response to cost cutting.

Acknowledgment that all departments of the hospital generated expenses that needed to be controlled resulted in across-the-board budget reduction. Throughout this era of health care history, the cost controls were departmentally driven, resulting in decreasing labor budgets but seldom changing the systems of work.

Concepts of quality management from industrial settings began to appear in hospital literature and the focus gradually shifted from cost control to problem solving with the expectation that hospital departments would identify their problems and solve them. The early efforts continued to be primarily departmentally driven. Recognition that high-quality patient care and successful expense control depended on collaboration among departments moved the problem-solving process into interdepartmental approaches.

New concerns about quality and impact on community health status again changed the focus, and the introduction of the concept of outcome measurement and management became prevalent. The goal of hospital leadership was redefined to managing processes of care cost-effectively while achieving desired outcomes.

Over the past seven years, the authors have been involved in Strengthening Hospital Nursing: A Program to Improve Patient Care. This program has provided the authors the opportunity to follow organizations as they institute changes in order to achieve their stated goals. Some of the profound changes that have occurred are described within the text of the chapters. The willingness of management to acknowledge that leadership is a shared accountability, and that leadership comes from many diverse locations in an organization when management opens the decision-making processes to all, was evident at all the grantees' sites. Transformational leadership speaks to creating a new organization that results in the alignment of personal, organizational, and community goals. When accomplished, everyone has achieved recognition as a valued individual, everyone has learned the skills of challenging and questioning the present reality, and everyone has the opportunity to take their place as leaders in order to build a stronger, more humanistic health care delivery system.

When the new collective leadership clarifies its vision, opens its doors to consumer input, and recognizes the value of holistic care, it will then begin to address the needs for ambulatory health care with the emphasis on wellness and prevention. This transition is currently under way and will require leadership to address the issues of wellness and prevention on a higher conceptual plane, exchanging single organization's benefit concept to a communitywide benefit. Leadership must create a collaborative model that builds on the valuable contribution that all community organizations should and can make for the community's welfare.

Transformational Leadership: Renewing Fundamental Values and Achieving New Relationships in Health Care provides the reader with insights on how managers are working toward this level of achievement in transforming leadership, thus transforming the systems of health care for the benefit of the people served.

Barbara A. Donaho, RN, MA, FAAN
Director, Strengthening Hospital Nursing Program

Acknowledgments

The authors would like to express thanks to Marshall Lucas, administrative assistant, SHNP National Program Office, for his consistent review of many versions of the manuscript and for his untiring support and constant and useful suggestions.

Thanks also are extended to SHNP project directors, codirectors, and other project staff, including evaluation and support staff, for attentiveness to multiple requests for information. They possess the "spirit" and energy needed for transformation described in this book. It is their belief, respect, and trust that often provided motivation to liberate leadership and organizational potentials to realize desired opportunities for patients and their families.

The authors would like to give special thanks to the Robert Wood Johnson Foundation and the Pew Charitable Trusts program, financial, and evaluation staffs and boards of trustees for their constant support and belief in the national program. With their commitment to finding new ways—the best ways—of bringing about a fundamental change in health care delivery, SHNP was able to demonstrate that care of patients can be strengthened through institutionwide collaborative efforts of all disciplines at all levels of an organization.

The authors would like to recognize the American Hospital Publishing staff for accepting the challenge of articulating transformation. Although the authors realize it takes the talent of many people working behind the scenes to publish a book, we particularly are grateful for the efforts and support of Brian Schenk, Richard Hill, Audrey Kaufman, and Linda Conheady. Of these individuals, we are especially grateful for Brian's vision and leadership. He believed that individuals who want to achieve an improved health care delivery system will benefit from the insights of those who have experienced the challenges and rewards of actual transformation of leadership styles.

Finally, the authors would like to thank patients, their families, and the communities served by those leaders and organizations represented in this book; it is for them that we have learned to be attentive to the soul of our institutions and all stakeholders and have formed new relationships to realize opportunities in achieving value-driven outcomes and fulfill our personal and organizational destiny.

Introduction

The concepts presented throughout this book are related to the role of leaders in transforming an organization to:

- Deliver improved value
- Identify and realize opportunities
- Form new and improved existing relationships
- Align with its destiny
- Care for its soul

Although there are many processes that organizations can use to transform operations, this book does not espouse any particular method of change. Transformed organizations have similar experiences and common outcomes regardless of the change method used.

The authors have been fortunate in having outstanding health care leaders, including those in the national program Strengthening Hospital Nursing: A Program to Improve Patient Care (SHNP), an initiative jointly sponsored by the Robert Wood Johnson Foundation and the Pew Charitable Trusts, participate in the writing of this book as contributors. Chief executive officers, chief operating officers, chief financial officers, nurse executives, and other hospital and health care system executive leaders and consultants from many areas, including information systems and human resources, share personal experiences within their institutions and communities. Board of trustee members provide insights from experiences with change processes and offer opinions regarding new responsibilities as a result of those processes. Physicians comment on their "Ah ha" experiences and how their role or attitude changed with involvement in interactive and interdisciplinary processes. Their comments and observations illustrate the principles and applications of transformational leadership. It is the wealth of experience represented by these leaders, presented within the framework of actual transformation of a variety of institutions using a wide spectrum of change processes, that forms the basis of this book.

Sharing in the experience of persons who have participated in this kind of transformation is highly instructive in moving from concept to practical application. Many report the change process itself has been the major factor in preparing to meet the demands of health care reform, especially in downsizing, mergers, and other cost reduction activities.

SHNP project directors provide rich insight into their successes and failures during transformation and articulate the why, how, and importance of building relationships with all persons throughout a wide continuum of health care. Contributors share how collaborative partnerships with employees, payers, policymakers, unions, and the community result in accomplishing their desired future, a future that is better for the whole health care system, not just individual members. With cocreators, they use visioning to define a philosophy of care that values patient-centeredness — that is, delivery of services designed to meet the needs of patients and their families rather than those of a department, care setting, or discipline. Leaders agree that the status quo no longer is acceptable, financial success no longer is an end point, mistakes can be acknowledged and celebrated as learning opportunities, and the organization is only as effective as its people. Transformational leaders make a principal investment in people as cocreators.

Poor flexibility, slow responsiveness, inadequate patient needs–response focus, preoccupation with activity rather than outcomes, bureaucratic paralysis, lack of innovation, and persistence of competition are prevalent in the health care system today. Transformational leaders are needed to reengineer the system. In *Reengineering the Corporation* Hammer and Champy write: "Reengineering is the fundamental rethinking and radical redesign of our business processes to achieve dramatic improvements in critical, contemporary measures of performance, such as cost, quality, and service."[1] Reengineering is not downsizing or a quick fix; rather, it is starting over. It is rethinking human resources, financial performance, and technological management, including operational and clinical systems. It is asking the question again and again: "Why are we doing this in the first place?"

Anxiety and discontent are common emotions as we absorb and reflect on the daily news and see the ways we relate to each other and to our world, especially in current attempts at major reform in the health care, welfare, and ecological systems. A large opportunity exists not only between what we are and what we would like to be, but also between what we presently are doing and what we should be doing. We would like to narrow the range of opportunities, if not fully realize them. A leader in this type of transformation should be able to motivate and energize followers to make a continuing analysis of personal, organizational, and societal opportunities, and to inspire them to work for desired outcomes that will benefit them, their organization, and their society simultaneously.

The transformational leader provides a clear role model and stimulus for others to identify and realize opportunities in personal and organizational life. Transformational leadership includes a spiritual dimension to recognize and honor the essence, or soul, of persons and their organizations in seeking to harmonize and heal the current divisions that threaten us. Moore says that "soul" is difficult to define, because to do so is an intellectual exercise, and soul manifests itself more through the imagination than through the intellect.[2] Soul has to do with genuineness and depth, and is revealed in attachments and relationships, not only with others but also with self and the environment.

The ability to care for, and to teach others to care for, the soul in each other and in our organization is the single most important attribute that leaders need to create responsive, adaptable, synergistic organizations, including a holistic health care system for the future. Honoring the soul of each other, of self, of organization, and of community correctly aligns and energizes all involved in a transformational process. Kaiser says that the transformational leader "alters organizational reality by hearing the call of destiny and volunteering to be a channel for its outworking."[3]

Transformational leadership builds on a base of sound business principles and common sense. It adds new concepts of value and destiny to the old paradigms of economics and competition. In defining *value*, it can be said that improved quality yields increased value and lower cost represents greater value. Moore says that:

> Soulful businesses are run differently in terms of profits, profit-sharing, ethics, attitudes towards the environment, and relationships to the communities in which they live; the soul life of this country is dependent on the economics also being soulful. If the economics do not have these values, then the country won't either. Soul in business is a major piece of the whole fabric. . . . If we're not willing to press beneath the bottom line, then we don't have a chance as a society."[4]

Organizations that recognize and honor the soul of the business add value for their customers and fulfill their destiny. Corporate and personal goals are aligned and aggressive financial targets are tempered with harmony, honesty, trust and compassion. Emphasis on competition is moderated by cooperation, collaboration, and cocreation. Traditional measures of corporate wealth are changed; financial assets derived from productivity and profit are broadened to include community responsibility, social accountability, and personal fulfillment of employees.[5]

References

1. Hammer, M., and Champy, J. *Reengineering the Corporation: A Manifesto for Business Revolution.* New York City: HarperCollins Publishers, 1993.

2. Moore, T. *Care of the Soul.* New York City: HarperCollins Publishers, 1992.

3. Kaiser, L. R. The visionary manager. In: T. C. Wilson, editor. *Emerging Issues in Health Care 1988.* Estes Park, CO: Estes Park Institute, 1988, pp. 94–104.

4. Infusino, D. The reluctant guru. *American Way* 27(12):70–112, June 15, 1994.

5. Ray, M., and Rinzler M. *The New Paradigm in Business: Emerging Strategies for Leadership and Organizational Change.* New York City: Jeremy P. Tarcher/ Perigee Books, 1993.

Part One

Setting the Stage for Organizational Change

• Introduction to Part 1

The split between what is nourishing at work and what is agonizing is the very chasm from which our personal destiny emerges. Accepting the presence of this chasm we can begin to deal, one step at a time, with the continually hidden, underground forces that shape our lives, often against our will. . . . Institutions must now balance the need to make a living with a natural ability to change. They must honor the souls of the individuals who work for them and the great soul of the natural world from which they take their resources.

The Heart Aroused: Poetry and the Preservation of the Soul in Corporate America, David Whyte

The keys to successful organizational change are flexibility, innovation, and adaptability. An organization's ability to change depends in large part on the willingness of its people—both leaders and staff—to take risks and to extend both personal and organizational boundaries. Although managing change is extremely difficult, the initial step of motivating an organization to change can be even more challenging. Typically, organizational change is motivated by a combination of forces: The organization is pushed to grow by a dissatisfaction with the current reality and pulled by the obvious desirability of improving value. Motivation to change also can be stimulated by the excitement of defining opportunities that are shared by all the organization's stakeholders.

According to Bennis, the work force of the near future will be characterized by higher levels of education and job mobility.[1] People will be "other oriented," and will take cues for values and norms from the immediate environment rather than past patterns and traditions. As a result, greater involvement, participation, and autonomy will be required in the workplace. Leaders will be confronted with enormous challenges, including the need to:

- Maintain control and yet still give people the freedom and autonomy they need to do their work
- Bring out the resourcefulness and creativity of the work force and yet maintain cost efficiency
- Develop habits of effectiveness that avoid quick-fix and short-term thinking and still manage turbulence and uncertainty

One response to change is for leaders to develop principles, beliefs, and values that stakeholders throughout the organization can accept. In his book *Principle-Centered Leadership,* Covey tells leaders to "get principles at the center of your life, your relationships, your management structures, and at the center of your organization."[2] These principles should operate regardless of the environment or prevailing market condition. Rather than lean on traditional patterns of power, status, or credentials, leaders who have defined a principle-centered style should influence and lead others through trust, sincerity, integrity, respect, and honor, which increase their ability to achieve an otherwise unattainable outcome. Such leaders are *transformational leaders*—individuals who are able to imagine alternatives for the future of their organizations and to adapt to the tension between what is and what is not controllable. Instead of responding defensively by becoming rigid and immobilized, transformational leaders are able to initiate processes for coping and to adjust to change in a prospective and proactive manner. They pay attention to the environment they serve,[3,4] understanding that: "To value oneself and, at the same time, to subordinate oneself to higher purposes and principles are the paradoxical essence of highest humanity and the foundation of effective leadership."[5]

Part 1 of this book consists of two chapters. Chapter 1, Defining the Forces for Change, identifies the current forces that many organizations feel are compelling them to change. Chapter 2, Recognizing the Benefits of Change, describes the characteristics of organizations that have realized the benefits of having made a successful transformation and identifies the qualities that characterize successful transformational leaders.

References

1. Bennis, W. *An Invented Life, Reflections on Leadership and Change.* Reading, MA: Addison-Wesley Publishing Co., 1993.

2. Covey, S. R. *Principle-Centered Leadership.* New York City: Simon & Schuster, 1992.

3. Kaiser, L. R. The visionary manager. In: T. C. Wilson, editor. *Emerging Issues in Health Care 1988.* Estes Park, CO: Estes Park Institute, 1988, pp.94–104.

4. Whyte, D. *The Heart Aroused: Poetry and the Preservation of the Soul in Corporate America.* New York City: Doubleday, 1994.

5. Covey.

Chapter 1

Defining the Forces for Change

> The most important force in health care revolution is a strong grass-roots movement of individuals and newly formed organizations dissatisfied with the existing system.
>
> *The Turning Point: Science, Society, and the Rising Culture,* Fritjof Capra

The major forces influencing health care reform are the increasing demands for quality and cost improvement, patient and community focus, effective resource management, and systems collaboration and integration. These demands stem from more than a mere imbalance in the law of supply and demand; rather, they represent an adjustment to the essence of the health care system itself, especially in terms of its relationship to the community.

This chapter discusses the forces that are bringing about organizational transformation and describes the qualities that characterize transformational leaders. It also includes the perspectives of a number of transformational leaders on the need to change.

• Quality and Cost Improvement

The public, including both patients and payers, is demanding value from health care providers. Improved quality, better service, and reduced cost are attributes of health care value. Health care administrators, providers, regulators, payers, and policymakers, as well as patients and their families, all have a role in the stewardship of providing higher value. Proper stewardship will result if the organization can define its destiny and if the organization's stakeholders can align with that destiny. The organization that can accomplish this will not only survive, it will prosper. However, in order for alignment to occur, unit-level staff as well as executive leaders and managers must feel personal responsibility for improving services. Each member of the organization should own the organizational vision and be recognized for his or her contribution toward improving the value of patient service. Additionally, each should understand who the customer is and should recognize that leadership and staff are customers to each other.

In the past decade, many ideas and conceptual frameworks have been developed for the management of health care quality and cost, including quality assurance, total quality management, and continuous quality improvement. If quality initiatives result in micromanagement solely for top-down cost-cutting outcomes rather than for institutionwide improvement of value, endorsed and practiced by everyone, it is likely that they will neither produce lasting efficiency outcomes nor sustain themselves over time. Often organizations embrace strategies without considering the long-term consequences as leaders look for quick fixes that will produce immediate cost reduction results. A more appropriate perspective is that of achieving long-range community outcomes such as reconfiguring the type of work force needed to meet specific community health demands or defining the requirements of an integrated health delivery system across a local community continuum of care.

Quality Improvement Initiatives Using a Unifying Theme

Many organizations undergoing effective transformation have integrated quality (value) improvement and management with clinical and operational innovations by using a single theme to identify the primary function of institutionwide programs. Examples of such institutions and the themes they have adopted include:

- Providence Portland Medical Center, Portland, Oregon, and its program titled Redesign and Improvement of Care Delivery, used the trajectory model to develop a new and improved delivery system that is continuous, flexible, and responsive to patient and family needs across care environments including acute care, home care, long-term care, and preventive care. The concept of patient outcomes, measurement, and use of date for clinical and operational decision making are key components of their redesign efforts (discussed later in this chapter).
- Beth Israel Hospital, Boston, and its program titled Integrated Clinical Practice, resulted in the redesign of nursing roles to improve utilization and integration of professional and technical staff into their work environments; in the design of a Clinical Entry Nurse Residency program to integrate new graduate nurses into a fast-paced teaching hospital; in the design of systems of care, focusing on the shift to ambulatory and community settings, and their integration with existing systems; and in the integration of patients' needs into work redesign efforts.

- Abbott-Northwestern Hospital, Minneapolis, and its program titled INNO-VATION, built upon the shared vision that "Patients are the reason we exist and people are the reason we excel." The guiding principles for INNOVATION are: work is patient driven, relationships are at the core of every interaction, and innovation creates ways to simplify systems. Specific projects include: bridging the care delivery continuum, reengineering information systems, implementing collaborative governance for nurses and other health professionals, redesigning the nursing education department into a center for education, and restructuring inpatient care units.
- Northeast Health Consortium, Rockland, Maine, and its program titled Northeast Health Consortium for Integrated Care System, designed a case management model of care delivery that allows nurses and other health professionals to manage the care of patients and their families across care settings, including acute care, home care, and long-term care.
- District of Columbia General Hospital, Washington, DC, and its program titled Patient-Centered Care Delivery System, initiated professional development efforts for nurses and other health care professionals, incorporated patient focus groups to learn from the patient how to improve services, designed collaborative care project teams that support the coordination of care at unit levels by interdisciplinary teams, and improved relationships with the Washington, DC area schools of nursing.
- University Hospitals/Pennsylvania State University at the Milton S. Hershey Medical Center, Hershey, Pennsylvania, and its program titled HORIZONS — Partnerships in Patient Care, designed a collaborative management model that facilitates relationship building between clinical and operational staff, and involves physicians, nurses, and other health care professionals. The objectives of HORIZONS including developing a system of patient care that incorporates the input and experiences of all stakeholders, including patients and their families to improve care outcomes; developing a high quality work environment, and designing a budget neutral, cost effective system of care delivery.

The mission, values, and vision of these organizations serve as the foundation for each of these programs. Each institution has designed an education program that will ensure that everyone in the organizational transformation fills his or her role in a consistent and constant manner. From top-level management to unit and support staff, everyone is accountable for clinical and operational improvement. These programs have shifted from individual accountability to team accountability, recognizing that the collective "we" brings the most effective result. To accomplish this team approach, a common process has been developed for identifying the differences in current reality and desired outcomes. Common language is used throughout the institution, and data collection methods and assessment indicators are defined before implementation begins. Data are collected based on the defined indicators to determine the effectiveness of outcomes. All aspects of the process and implementation are documented in a notebook, forming a charter that is presented to each team starting an innovation process.

Quality Plans That Establish Integration between Medical Staff and Hospital Staff Accountability

Integration of a common process for medical staff and institutional staff quality improvement activities results in joint accountability for efficacious and appropriate patient care services. These plans shift the focus of performance from the individual and the department to key functions throughout the entire organization, emphasizing team accountability. Key functions might include, for example, patient assessment, patient-centered treatment, physician and employee education on new technology, organizational performance improvement, information management, medical staff development, quality control, and patient, physician, and employee satisfaction. These quality plans are based on a philosophy of patient-centeredness that views patient care processes as part of a continuum that provides patients and their families access to an integrated system of settings, services, and care levels. Input from physicians, nurses, utilization review, finance, social service, education, information systems, and pastoral care provides the necessary expertise for adapting elements of the plan to the practices of each discipline. The end result is an interdisciplinary process that includes persons from all levels of management, is approved by both medical staff and board of trustees, and is disseminated as the institutionwide plan based on delivering value demanded by the community (health care public).

However, no quality improvement plan or management strategy will achieve maximal success unless it provides meaning to the people who implement it. When the organizational mission is congruent with the employee's personal goals, shared responsibility and shared leadership for improving services for patients and their families are more likely to exist. It is the transformational leader's responsibility to provide employees the opportunity to do more than bring home a paycheck. Employees want to believe in their work. They want work that can excite them when they start their day. They seek responsibilities that give them energy and that are worthwhile for the common purpose.[1-4]

• Patient and Community Focus

Universal health care coverage, adequate access to treatment, overall cost containment, and quality improvement are defined and articulated challenges for building healthier communities.[5] Health policy change and financial reform, though essential, are not enough to meet these challenges alone. If patient and community demands are to be met, the relationships between hospital-based services and other care settings, including home care, wellness care, long-term care, rehabilitative care, and other community- or neighborhood-based services, also must be redefined. The ability of health care executive leadership and boards of trustees to recognize the importance of the integrated relationships between care settings is the first step in designing a responsive continuum of care. The external and internal forces affecting the organization, the characteristics of leadership and managers, the mission and values of the organization, and the strategic direction based on its vision are factors that influence how the organization will respond to these demands.

Consumers and purchasers of health care usually do not accurately assess the technical quality of health services; rather, they perceive the human dimensions of care such as empathy, responsiveness, reliability, communication, and caring.[6] Thus, organizations that pay attention to how and where health care is delivered play a stronger role in their communities. Developing operational definitions and specifying levels of performance for the human dimensions of care enhances development of community-focused relationships. Following are examples of two service delivery systems that were designed to respond to the needs of specific communities.

The Patient-Centered Care Delivery System

District of Columbia General Hospital (DCGH), Washington, DC, is located in a socially and economically deprived area within a neighborhood known for a high crime rate. DCGH implemented the patient-centered care delivery system (PCCDS), defined by institutional stakeholders as "health care and hospital services designed to place the primary focus on meeting the individualized patient needs through a multidisciplinary approach." DCGH leaders believe that "a patient-centered hospital is achieved with the proper skills, knowledge, and attitudes that allow harmonious work in a diverse workforce within a diverse community, and patient-centered care is everyone's business."[7]

All employees, administrators, and care providers at all levels, including physicians, are involved in meeting patient care services in a timely and efficient manner in the appropriate setting. For the hospital, this means addressing both wellness and health education as part of the service system. Mark Chastang, former chief executive officer (CEO), indicates that early in DCGH's change process, high-quality care with attention on financial constraints was the motivating factor for the system. After a hospital retreat, he and his leadership team formulated strategies for patient-centered care and placed them into the hospital strategic plan. That plan, and the vision for a patient-centered hospital, was endorsed by hospital commissioners and medical staff who were actively involved in its development.

Through patient, family, and employee focus groups, hospital leadership learned that DCGH was not perceived in its service area as caring, responsive, safe, clean, or efficient. In fact, in 1990, one woman said: "We come here only to die or when we are really sick, not to receive quality care." Patient perceptions about the lack of caregiver interest and long waiting times, along with limited expectations for high-quality care, became the motivating force behind the shift from the traditional department-driven model to patient-centered care.

Consultants from the Center for Applied Research, in Philadelphia, guided DCGH through organizational development processes for PCCDS using interactive planning and system thinking principles. Nurse consultants from the Center for Case Management in South Natick, Massachusetts, assisted them with elements of their collaborative patient care model. Educational, technical, and financial support from the Strengthening Hospital Nursing program (SHNP) provided them means and resources to realize their goal of PCCDS.

Without the enthusiasm and dedication of Chastang and Nellie Robinson, previous associate administrator for nursing, and without the project staff's energy and dedication to project details, this vision would not have been achieved. Their trust and obvious respect for each person's contribution were the compelling forces behind the project's success. During one SHNP site visit, Chastang said, "What I've done, perhaps more than anything else, is *to listen* to competent, creative, and motivated staff and *to encourage* each of them to lead. There is an expectation that all employees, not just administration, are masters of our change."

Hallmarks of the PCCDS are:

- *Teams (collaborative care project teams)* including physicians, nurses, and other care providers working together to develop clinical pathways and other case management strategies for specific patient services.
- *Education* for care providers and support departments, including quality improvement, patient-centered care, guest relations, grand rounds, safety and security strategies and updates, and word processing.
- *Research* to monitor and assess effectiveness.
- *Management information systems* to integrate clinical financial, and customer satisfaction data.
- *Recognition activities* for everyone involved. Through the recognition program, both individual and collective successes for PCCDS are celebrated.

Caregiver Workshops

Another service delivery system designed to meet the needs of a specific patient population within the community was initiated by the Northeast Health Consortium, which comprises an acute care hospital, home care, and long-term care in the mid-coastal region of rural Maine. Responding to the needs of its growing elderly population, the Consortium developed a series of caregiver workshops. Susan Neves, geriatric facilitator for the Integrated Care Project, states: "There is a great need to give more attention to the elderly as that population group is growing, and most of these people and their families do not have the financial resources to purchase preventive or wellness services. The elderly rely on the support and care they can get from family and friends. Often family members are working and cannot get away during the day. This compounds the need to have the kind of classes we are offering." The workshops are presented in the evening for the convenience of those attending. They are intended to assist family and friends who often are suddenly thrust into the role of caregiver for an elderly loved one. The series provides the tools needed to meet the challenges of making caregiving choices that are best for all concerned. The workshops include stress management, aging and health, community resources, the how-to's of personal care, communication skills, and financial and legal decision making. The instructors include nurses, physical therapists, social workers, and others from community agencies. Transformational leaders will implement new services, such as these workshops, to reduce utilization by a capitated population or a population of patients that have their services prepaid.

• Resource Management

Resource management is another of the major forces bringing about change in health care delivery. Examples of effective resource management in hospitals undergoing successful transformation to patient-centered care include resource pooling, work and role redesign, and innovative information systems redesign.

Resource Pooling

One effective resource management strategy is resource pooling. In this strategy, hospitals in a region that are experiencing shortages in personnel and/or specialty equipment combine their talents and competencies. The need is especially acute among rural hospitals because they often have greater difficulty recruiting professional staff and staying up-to-date with advanced technology. One such collaboration that has proved successful is the Vermont Nursing Initiative (VNI), a consortium formed for the purpose of the SHNP. Committed to providing services to patients and their families within their own communities, the VNI designed and implemented the Staffing Network of the Rural Resource Pool. This voluntary registry includes nursing, pharmacy, physical therapy, medical records, X-ray technicians, and others and enables hospitals to share staff, equipment, and services in order to:

- Meet the professional and technical support staff needs of hospitals
- Prevent unnecessary transfers of patients out of their home hospital
- Provide appropriate specialty services for patients within their community

The collaboration has benefited hospitals, staff, and patients in many ways. For example, an X-ray technician in one of the smaller hospitals requested a much-earned vacation. In the past, this technician could take only a few days at a time because no competent cross-trained personnel was available within the institution to fill in for her. However, with the new resource pool, a colleague from another hospital could take over her responsibilities in her absence. This sharing of resources allowed the technician extended time away, maintained X-ray department services, and strengthened a collaborative relationship between the two hospitals. In another example, a patient requiring a surgical procedure previously might have been transferred because the admitting hospital did not have a surgical assistant for the physician. The VNI designed a surgical first assistant program for nurses that allowed a pool of nurses with special training to assist physicians for specific procedures, making patient transfer unnecessary.

Work and Role Redesign

Other institutions are combining work and role redesign and restructuring with reengineering strategies to create new roles or design new ways for people to work together. Similar to the VNI strategies, such strategies enhance the skill definition needed by caregivers for specific patient services, clarify roles for professionals, and differentiate the uniqueness of their contribution to patient care outcomes. These strategies also provide a mechanism for defining accountability for patient care outcomes and a means for justifying support staff. They help ensure that the patient's needs are met by the most appropriate care provider.

Most institutions that have completed a successful transformation to patient-centered care realize that role or job restructuring should come only once the work is defined. An organization committed to a patient-centered delivery system will define the work and the roles needed to carry out that work by defining the specific needs of the patient. However, if the organization is driven only by the needs of departments or the financial bottom line, work and roles will be defined according to those driving forces. Using these new strategies, hospital managers and interdisciplinary teams have worked together to change the skill mix of specific unit-level staff, which has resulted in cost efficiencies and more appropriate use of professional care providers. For example, a rehabilitation unit will manage patient care efficiently with a higher ratio of technical staff to professional staff, whereas a critical care unit will require a higher ratio of professional staff to manage more intensely ill patients. In addition to sustaining and improving value, both units have patient services met by the person most appropriate to provide the service. Not only is the skill mix changed, but working relationships and how the work gets done also are changed. Moreover, to be effective, work and role redesign efforts must involve those individuals whose work or role will be affected. This will require that multidisciplinary teams work together to develop and implement the new roles.

Work and role redesign affects both professional and support workers. The *professional worker* may be defined as a caregiver using cognitive skills and practicing under the policies of a specific license. As a result of work and role redesign, new roles are emerging for professional workers, ranging from advanced practitioners managing the care of patients across settings (integrated clinical practice) to differentiated roles of unit-level nurses, such as nurse case managers, clinical managers, care coordinators, and others. Collaborative management triads composed of a nurse, a physician, and an administrator are evolving as a new management system within inpatient and outpatient settings, as well as in nurse-managed settings. Clinical nurse specialist roles often are more broad based, allowing the specialist to function across settings within not only the hospital but also the community. Roles for nurse practitioners are developing in nontraditional settings such as emergency departments (EDs), critical care areas, and other specialty units. Some nurse practitioners are collaborating with attending physicians to manage certain patient groups, often assuming the provider functions of residents in teaching hospitals where the supply of residents is limited.

Support worker roles also are evolving as professionals delegate tasks that are suited to their practice and effectively meet the needs of patients and families. The *support worker* is defined as someone who is responsible for repetitive tasks under the direction of a licensed professional. Often the support worker role is multifunctional, multiskilled, or multicompetent. Support functions that can be combined satisfactorily are clerical, housekeeping, transport, and admissions. Technical skills that often are combined include dietary, respiratory, physical therapy, clinical laboratory, and nursing.

Thus, within the framework of patient-centered care, both professional and support staff are changing to meet the needs of patients and their families in the most appropriate setting. Many have the potential for cutting across a variety of service settings, allowing for improved productivity of the worker, enhanced continuity of care for the patient, and cost savings for the organization. (These concepts are discussed in greater detail in the book *Work and Role Redesign: Tools and Techniques for the Health Care Setting* by Ruth B. Hanson and Betty Sayers.[8])

Innovative Information Systems Redesign

A third strategy for effective resource management is innovative information systems redesign. During a networking meeting for information systems (IS), representatives from 40 SHNP institutions discussed the role of IS in an organization dealing with change, specifically in relation to a PCCDS that is based on continuity of care integrated across all care settings. In discussing their role as meaningful contributors to the enhancement of their organizations' missions, the representatives identified several improvements. These included an integrated medical record that would move electronically across care settings and link physician offices and eventually the homes of patients and their families; user interfaces both within and outside the hospital; prototypes for new applications; and global networking capabilities to share information. Information systems are of critical importance in the restructuring, redesign, and reengineering process with increasing need for data and data analysis, trending, and monitoring. Additionally, it is important for establishing collection points for clinical information at the bedside and support areas. These functions are enhanced, facilitated, and managed by a well-integrated IS department, and the organization of the future may be only as efficient as its IS allows it to be. The communication highway is electronically paved and will serve as the most efficient mechanism for linking care settings with a master community medical index containing specific clinical service and quality data repositories.

Report cards to rate providers on clinical outcomes and customer satisfaction are an expectation of payers, employers, and government. Quality indicators already are used by managed care purchasers to evaluate and determine provider selection. Successful health care networks will form an integrated IS to allow care providers to have reliable and accurate clinical and cost data in real time at the point of care. This will be the basis for timely, consistent, and accurate data for report cards.

Conventionally, information management has been driven by the work of the organization resulting in an IS network that is aligned with management processes, individual skills, and the technology required to provide service and support to users. Future applications may warrant an entirely different approach, as noted in the summer 1994 issue of *Sloan Management Review*. Rather than begin with business strategy, this process of design begins with the tactical and incremental adoption of information technology solely to meet current operational needs.[9] This approach generates a range of new strategic options that otherwise would not surface. The process is grounded in systems thinking and organizational learning.

All resources will have to be managed differently, considering the needs of patients and their families while innovating or sustaining value. As Barbara Donaho, director of SHNP, has observed: "Resource management is only as good as the people in the organization who understand and implement processes for improved value."

• System Collaboration and Integration

The final major force influencing change in health care delivery is system collaboration and integration. Alliances between providers and payers are becoming a necessity for survival in the process of health care reform. These relationships must yield benefits to both parties and must evolve progressively beyond the initial reason for integration to allow maximum opportunities and options to develop. Successful alliances involve collaboration and cocreation. Synergistically, they create new value rather than merely return results equal to the individual investments. The talents, knowledge, and skills that each party brings to the desired outcome are valued. These relationships cannot be controlled in the traditional manner, but must be built on interpersonal and interorganizational trust with a sound, yet adaptable infrastructure.

As an example, Providence Portland Medical Center involved payers in the implementation of its redesign and improvement of care delivery program. Using a trajectory model, the medical center developed a new and improved patient needs–responsive delivery system. The model's goal is care provision that is "continuous, flexible, responsive to what the ill person requires, and it is respectful of the ill person and their families."[10] Marie Driever, co-project director for the center's SHNP project, describes it as follows:

> The trajectory model is based on the assumption that the home is the primary place where illness is managed on a daily basis. In the face of illness, the ill person and the family seek to maintain quality of life. The work of the care professional is only one part of the overall management of the patient. The effectiveness of the health care professional's work is judged on two dimensions: its technical quality and its "fit" with the needs of the patient and the family. From the assumptions, it becomes apparent that other players must be involved, or satisfactory patient care outcomes cannot be achieved. For example, our rehabilitation and obstetrics services have both negotiated new reimbursement mechanisms with third-party insurers to support out-of-hospital services for their patient populations. For Providence, this is a breakthrough and we are excited as we seek to advance their work to other patient groups.

The Northeast Health Care Consortium also developed a new relationship with payers. A member facility, Penobscot Bay Medical Center, developed an outpatient program for care of children with asthma. Designed and implemented by the pediatric and ED nursing and medical staff, the program demonstrates that care is more efficacious and appropriate if it is given by the parent in the home setting. Improved patient outcomes demonstrate improved quality of cost-efficient care for the child. This program has a

high value for everyone involved, including payers. Parent and child education, wellness care, and preventive management are now reimbursed, along
with traditional emergency and acute care. According to Paula Delahanty,
the center's director of quality management, the program is a great success:
"Children feel so much better if they can be cared for by Mom and go to
school with their friends . . . They are learning how to live with their asthma
differently, and emergency visits have greatly decreased."

• Transformational Leaders on the Need for Change

Following are the perspectives of various transformational leaders on the
need for change in health care. Their observations also underscore their role
in the change process.

*George Belsey, chairman and CEO, Air Methods Corporation (form-
erly of the American Hospital Association):* To survive, hospitals must cut
costs and learn how to bear financial risk. Becoming part of an organization larger than themselves is critical. There will be no room in the future
for redundant tests, unnecessary procedures, and the expense associated with
overutilization of the system. The incentives of a capitated system will go
a long way to ameliorate this problem. This means managed care will reduce
the flow of patients to the traditional hospital. That is desirable if the hospital
is a part of a system and functioning as a cost center. The hospital becomes
the center for highly specialized services — more of a referral center than a
place patients go to for care because of its convenient neighborhood location or "where they've always gone." An article in the January 10, 1994, issue
of *Barron's* points out that in the future, "a hospital's market share will be
assessed not by how many patients doctors funnel through its doors, but
by the renewal rate of its contracts with managed care companies. . . . A
hospital operator who thinks of his or her institution as an acute care center,
delivering medical care and performing surgeries, is headed for Jurassic
Park; . . . the hospital is, instead, becoming a base for technology that might
be delivered in someone's home, at a rehab center or an alternative site."

Hospitals that rethink inefficient processes capitalize on technology, cut
costs, and function as a part of an integrated delivery system. A study by
Arthur D. Little Company stated that hospitals could save $36 billion a year
on health care through advanced information technologies including electronic billing and insurance claim filing, bedside computer terminals, on-
line patient records, diagnostic software, and telemedicine. On the reengineering front, we are seeing hospitals restructure services around patients by moving therapy centers to patient floors and training staff to work as teams.
Also, some hospitals are looking at performance-based contracts with outside vendors. Payment of vendors will be determined to a significant extent
on patient impressions about services during their stay, including dietary

and housekeeping. Exceptional providers of care in the future will make a major emphasis in wellness programs. They will become heavily involved in their communities with such programs as prenatal care, health screenings, and exercise and smoking cessation classes. Over time, community outreach will enable them to deal with other social issues such as child abuse, domestic violence, housing, and education. In the last two decades, major emphasis has been placed on market share and revenue growth. For those institutions that would prefer the current rules, these changes will put them at great risk. For those institutions committed to trying to rationalize the use of resources and focus on the needs of their communities, these changes will be a welcome challenge.

Edward Foley, regional vice-president, Hospital Council of Southern California: As health care shifts over to a model that is consumer (patient) driven, rather than physician driven, employees and managers at all levels will accept and agree to changes that otherwise would not be realizable. Whether through the joy and satisfaction of excellent service to patients or out of fear of being a part of a nonviable organization, people will realize the need to participate in the transformation of their job and their organization. As patients slip into the driver's seat in health care delivery, resource managers (finance, human resources, information, technology, and others) will see the need and the wisdom of their own transformation, a transformation supportive of the organization's goal of patient responsiveness.

Nathan Stark, chairman of the SHNP National Advisory Committee: We excel on the technological side, but our system has fundamental flaws — high infant mortality and low life expectancy compared to other industrialized nations, costs consuming an incredible share of our gross national product, the lack of access to health care by millions, and the fear of being rendered destitute by millions more. The health of the American people is front and center on the American political stage. The stakes are too high — and the time too propitious — for more of the same old status quo.

Mark Burzynski, president and CEO, Yellowstone Community Health Plan (formerly CFO, Saint Vincent Hospital and Health Center, Billings, Montana, and the SHNP Project at the Montana Consortium for Excellence in Health Care): I have a responsibility to make a difference in three areas: (1) changing traditional attitudes, (2) participating in the development of networks and alternative delivery systems, and (3) implementing "social accountability." The CFOs of most organizations are uniquely positioned to make a difference. They traditionally are a "lonely voice" harping about expenses/cost management, FTEs, variance reports, etc., i.e., many things that are foreign to a clinician. Rather than teaching about resource management, we usually are micromanaging departments. Now, with a shift towards continuous improvement and attention on patient-focused care, CFOs have a new role as mentor and coach at the unit level or with departmental teams, teaching how to manage resources to do the right things for patients and their families. The CFO must believe that, if we really do the right things for the patient, the organization will be financially successful.

The second thing that the CFO must do is to change from a competitive attitude. Saint Vincent Hospital and Health Center (SVHHC) is a part of the Montana Consortium. A consortium by its nature should be a cooperative, collaborative venture and a vehicle for change. That, however, is not always the reality. Each member is burdened with biases, attitudes, beliefs and habits which interfere with the vision of an integrated network of hospitals. Collaboration is a part of our vocabulary; we read about it, but do we really know how to do it and actually have the guts to do it? I do not think so. In fact, I sometimes think the consortium would find it easier to work together if they had a "common opponent to defeat." We must let go of our outdated biases and attitudes and learn to know each others talents and competencies so that we can have at least "competitive collaboration." We must learn to trust and respect each other for what we bring to our common communities. Only through our belief in each other to do the right thing for the patient will we be able creatively to reengineer our financial systems to deal with the cost of services and form meaningful health care alliances.

Providing health care is a moral imperative. Success should be measured in terms of the health of the community. Alliances with physicians, payers, and the business community will be important factors as the hospital shifts from hospital-based care to a community-based system. SVHHC, in partnership with members of its medical staff, incorporated a physician–hospital organization, the Billings Physician Hospital Alliance, Inc. The alliance is a vehicle for contract arrangements. However, it has a deeper meaning in terms of building trust, rural hospital and physician linkages, and an educational forum where changes in the environment and in the health care industry are discussed. The trust and education fostered by the alliance are critical ingredients for a community health plan where the focus shifts to practice patterns.

I believe the role of a community health plan, such as YCHP, is to assist a community to achieve better health and to lower the risk to which high-risk individuals are vulnerable and which ultimately makes them uninsurable. I have challenges which focus on changing the behaviors and attitudes of care providers, as well as developing a new primary care model. It is apparent that effective managed care efforts and programs are not going to be based on contracts, payment levels, channeling mechanisms, utilization review, and quality assurance. Effectiveness will be based on relationships that providers can build between themselves and their community. Another goal is to develop a primary care clinic staffed by advanced practitioners who will do health assessments on high-risk patients who are uninsurable, and to design care plans for these patients in order to lower their risk factors over time. The intent is to facilitate their acceptance as an insurance risk. . . . [The YCHP] will act as an insurer as well as a provider, offer a vertically integrated health care system, be partners with and accountable to the community, and organize providers and the community into a nurturing support system. YCHP is the next phase of managed care, which takes our industry beyond discount medicine with limited access through authorization and medical underwriting, i.e., the concepts of preexisting conditions, "locking out uninsurables", and "cherry picking."

During the next phase of managed health care, providers will accept responsibility for the delivery of "value-based" care; care will be directed at those who need it, appropriate types and levels of care will be delivered, and providers will be accountable for the health status of a defined population. Restructured delivery systems, community orientation about services and support, attributes of patient-centeredness, and continuity of care through an integrated/seamless systems will be characteristics of the YCHP and others that are accepting health and social accountability for their communities.

• Conclusion

Organizational change should be considered if local forces are demanding improved value, reflected in higher quality and better service at lower cost. These forces include the need for quality and cost improvement, focus on patient and community needs, effective resource management, and recognition for expanding system collaboration and integration. All or any of these factors may be enough to push the organization to risk undergoing transformation by creating incentives to change hospital utilization patterns from inpatient to outpatient services, including wellness care and prevention care.

References

1. Stein, M., and Hollwitz, J. *Psyche at Work: Workplace Applications of Jungian Analytical Psychology.* Wilmette, IL: Chiron Publications, 1992.

2. Covey, S. R. *The 7 Habits of Highly Effective People: Powerful Lessons in Personal Change.* New York City: Simon & Schuster, 1990.

3. Senge, P. M., Roberts, C., Ross, R. B., Smith, B. J., and Kleiner, A. *The Fifth Discipline Fieldbook: Strategies and Tools for Building a Learning Organization.* New York City: Doubleday, 1994.

4. The Healthcare Forum Leadership Center's Healthier Communities Partnership. *Healthier Communities Action Kit: A Guide for Leaders Embracing Change.* Module 1. San Francisco: The Healthcare Forum, 1993.

5. *Bridging the Leadership Gap in Healthcare.* Executive Summary of a National Study conducted by the Leadership Center of the Healthcare Forum. San Francisco: The Healthcare Forum, 1992.

6. Bowers, M. R., Swan, J. E., and Koehler, W. F. What attributes determine quality and satisfaction with health care delivery. *Health Care Management Review* 19(4):49–55, Fall 1994.

7. Jacks, G., and Hunt, C. T. *Patient-Centered Care: Everyone's Business.* Washington, DC: District of Columbia General Hospital, 1994.

8. Hanson, R. B., and Sayers, B. *Work and Role Redesign: Tools and Techniques for the Health Care Setting.* Chicago: American Hospital Publishing, 1995.

9. Yetton, P. W., Johnston, K. D., and Craig, J. F. Computer-aided architects: a case study of IT and strategic change. *Sloan Management Review* 35(4):57–65, Summer 1994.

10. Providence Medical Center adopts trajectory model to deliver patient-focused care. *Strengthening* 1(3):2, 4, 8, Winter 1994.

Chapter 2

Recognizing the Benefits of Change

> Change efforts have to mobilize people around what is not yet known, not yet experienced . . . the architects of change have to operate on a symbolic as well as a practical level, choosing out all possible truths.
>
> *The Change Masters: Innovation and Entrepreneurship in the American Corporation,* Rosabeth Moss Kanter

The forces for change discussed in chapter 1 are negative factors that *push* an organization to change because of dissatisfaction with the current reality. Often they represent demands for change from the outside. This chapter considers the positive factors that *pull* an organization to change. These are the factors that may make transformation attractive enough to the organization's leaders and stakeholders that they will embrace change because of the improvements in value it can bring.

This chapter describes the characteristics of health care organizations that have successfully realized the benefits of change. It also discusses the characteristics of transformational leaders.

• Characteristics of Successful Health Care Organizations

Generally, health care organizations that have successfully negotiated change share certain characteristics. They:

- Are interdependent
- Seek value-driven outcomes
- Deliver patient-centered care
- Participate in a continuum of care

The following subsections describe these characteristics.

Successful Organizations Are Interdependent

Previously competing independent health care organizations now are cooperating to improve the health of their communities. Their relationship with each other usually moves from independence, through a stage of cautious collaboration, into true mutual interdependence, often with shared revenue and debt, as they become cocreators of community health networks. The organizational shift from independence to interdependence is mirrored in the individual relationships of the workforce as they learn to respect and rely on each other in new ways for the good of their patients.

These thriving, prosperous health care organizations have management approaches that encourage trust and show respect for the well-being of all stakeholders involved in a patient's care, including the patient, his or her family, and his or her care providers. The creativity, talent, knowledge, and skills of everyone involved in the health care of the community are valued, rewarded, and utilized appropriately as opportunities for improvement are identified and realized. Additionally, self-directed and self-reliant behaviors that respect others are supported by management and compensated with appropriate rewards and recognition.[1,2] Individuals from all levels of the organization demonstrate responsibility and behave in ways that show trust and respect for other staff members' work. They take pride in their work, in the work of the organization, and in the contribution the organization makes to the community. Management moves from centralized decision making to collaborative and interdependent behavior.[3-5]

Table 2-1 outlines three typical stages of organizational development and the behavioral characteristics of each stage. It is derived from observations made by SHNP staff and National Advisory Committee members during institution site visits, as well as from comments made by contributors to this book.

Successful Organizations Seek Value-Driven Outcomes

To survive in the current health care marketplace, a health care organization must seek value-driven outcomes. The desired value-driven outcome necessary for survival is improved quality at lower cost. Thus, organizational decision making should focus on alternatives or options that will achieve better value for the patient, his or her family, and the organization alike. Such decision making answers the question, What do we really want for our patients in this community? Answers are implemented in a systemwide approach to achieve the most desirable opportunities for improving organizational performance. One way to do this is to create a value framework (described in detail in chapter 4). A value framework allows executive leadership, boards of trustees, and everyone at all levels of the organization to develop a common language for understanding values. The value framework becomes a part of daily organizational operations, whether the work

Table 2-1. Stages of Organizational Development

Behaviors	Stage		
	Dependent	**Independent**	**Interdependent**
Decision making	Highly centralized	Decentralized, autonomous	Decentralized, but collaborative
Trust level	Low	Generally high	High
Maturity level	Low	Higher, with confidence in key staff displayed	High, with confidence, trust, and respect
Opportunity identification	Minimal	Inconsistent, usually project focused	Predictable and institutionalized
Management style	Autocratic	Encourages staff autonomy	Participative, partnerships and co-creators
Behavioral expectations	Obedience, limited empowerment	Individual performance	Collaborative teamwork and accountability

Adapted from R. Inguagiato, *Organizational Theory: Fundamentals of Medical Management* (Tampa: American College of Physician Executives, 1993); T. C. Cummings, and C. G. Worley, *Organization Development and Change* (St. Paul: West Publishing Company, 1993); and J. L. Gibson, J. M. Ivancevich, and J. H. Donnelly, Jr., *Organizations: Behavior, Structure, Process* (Burr Ridge, IL: Richard D. Irwin, Inc., 1994).

is a daily routine responsibility or a corporate strategic action. John Lathrop, director of Strategic Insights, says:

> It is interesting how much we gain by simply being clear about our values and the resulting performance goals. Once these are known, the organization can show those values to its customers, including patients and their families, suppliers, and care providers. Most importantly, decisions are made consistently, the institution works as a coherent system, and that consistency and coherence is focused on one desired outcome: effective and appropriate patient care.

The value framework allows freedom at every level, from senior management to unit staff, to make decisions pertaining to specific work while maintaining alignment within the whole organization.

Successful Organizations Deliver Patient-Centered Care

Successful health care organizations also deliver patient-centered care. *Patient-centeredness* is a philosophy of care focusing on the needs of the patient as the common goal of services and interventions provided by medical staff, clinicians, and management. In this philosophy, service delivery is designed to meet the needs of the patient and his or her family, rather than the needs of a department, care setting, or discipline. Patient-centeredness uses multiple clinical management methodologies, including managed care/case management, care paths (clinical pathways), and clinical protocols.

Successful Organizations Participate in a Continuum of Care

The successful health care system of the future is characterized as synergistic and interdependent, offering continuity of care throughout a spectrum of services in many settings. These settings include hospital-based care, home care, long-term care, maintenance care, preventive care, and wellness care — all within community locations that interrelate for ideal patient service outcomes. Whereas care services from such a synergistic system are effective, appropriate, and efficacious for the patient and his or her family, they also are enormously satisfying to care providers and leadership because they fulfill their personal and organizational goals. Leaders who provide input into this view of the health care system agree that cooperative and collaborative relationships are critical to a synergistic, interdependent system which embraces a seamless flow of service from one environment to another. Thus, the patient care delivery system is coordinated from the preadmission phase through the continuation or placement phase. The following subsections define these different phases.

Preadmission Phase

Preadmission is the process of initial assessment of the needs of the patient to determine the most appropriate care setting in the continuum of service. This phase includes linkages with:

- Physician offices and health care clinics/centers
- Other community care settings and agencies
- Acute care and specialty facilities
- Rehabilitation, long-term care, home care, and wellness care
- Maintenance care and prevention care, health promotions and education

Entry Phase

The entry phase is the determination of the appropriate provider resources required to deliver the greatest value. The entry phase includes:

- Determining appropriateness of level of care
- Determining availability of relevant services and interventions
- Making referral and transfer arrangements with other care settings

- Using outpatient, ambulatory, and maintenance services
- Determining availability of affiliate resources such as acute care facilities, home care, rehabilitation, skilled nursing facilities, and family medicine clinics
- Planning overall care, including placement and follow-up care

Intervention Phase

The continuous flow of care and services, from assessment through treatment and reassessment, is delivered in the intervention phase. This includes coordination of care among care providers, and involvement and education of the patient and family, wherever located within the continuum.

Preplacement Phase

Placement processes are planned and implemented with patient and family input during the preplacement phase. This component is a reevaluation of the appropriateness and efficacy of the plan of care, and includes provision of continuing care within care settings such as outpatient, subacute, long-term care, home care, rehabilitation, and wellness.

Continuation or Placement Phase

The placement phase includes activities related to the referral or transfer of the patient to other care settings, including home care, with appropriate follow-up or maintenance care services. Although this has been considered the discharge-from-the-hospital stage, it is important to note that the patient is not discharged from the system but, rather, remains in a different care setting within the continuum of care. Maintenance services can be provided in dedicated space within either a hospital or a clinic setting. Such services usually are given in a limited time frame and do not require 24-hour hospitalization.

• Characteristics of Transformational Leaders

The 1992 Healthcare Forum Leadership Center National Study titled Bridging the Leadership Gap in Healthcare indicated that future leaders need competencies different from their predecessors, with increased emphasis on personal and professional values. The leaders of the future will have to deal with the driving forces of change—economic, demographic, technological, environmental, political, and social—while striving to create a community-based system for services. The term used in this study to describe this change in approach is *transformational leadership.*[6]

Thus, transformational leaders are individuals who identify and achieve opportunities for improved consumer value and for building collegial relationships in partnerships. They inspire others in their quest for personal and organizational fulfillment by asking questions, setting direction, and managing the boundaries of the organization's business while liberating caregivers and other stakeholders to do their work. In his book *Leadership Is,* Owen writes: "To manage is to control; to lead is to liberate."[7] Creativity, imagination, and a participative management style that models and encourages collaborative staff behavior throughout the organization are skills used by transformational leaders. These individuals are achievers, yet place the well-being of others and the organization above personal endeavors.

Aggregated comments from health care executives show similar characteristics and values attributed to true transformational leaders. They indicate that transformational leaders:

- Are proactive and prospective
- Are charismatic and passionate
- Use noncensored communication
- Use self properly
- Are champions for change, politicians, and negotiators
- Are stewards
- Are contemplative
- Care for the souls of individuals and the organization
- Have integrity and respect colleagues
- Are catalysts for creativity and innovation
- Are facilitators
- Function as team members
- Practice personal learning and encourage organizational learning
- Are people centered
- Use holistic approaches
- Empower others
- Recognize that relationships are vital to restructuring and transition
- Often are cantadoras, or tellers of stories

Leaders Are Proactive and Prospective

One particularly valuable characteristic of transformational leaders is the ability to respond quickly and appropriately to the needs of the organization, the community, and society at large. Such leaders are driven by values rather than emotions. They take the initiative, anticipate, empathize, and often compensate for the limitations of others or the organization. They are considered advocates for strategic organizational adaptation. They are attentive to the future, yet learn from the past. In their book *Strategic Choices for America's Hospitals,* Shortell, Morrison, and Friedman indicate that prospective organizations and their leaders respond rapidly to early signals of market needs and opportunities, and consistently attempt to be the first to provide service to meet those needs.[8]

Leaders Are Charismatic and Passionate

Transformational leaders are dynamic individuals who use their creativity and imagination to achieve positive change by developing the skills and talents of others who have the passion to move the organization toward a defined future. Thus, the true transformational leader thinks in terms of doing what should be done for the good of the organization and the community, rather than in terms of personal recognition and reward. Senge and his colleagues point out that a leader cannot rely solely on personal power to influence; rather, his or her charisma must come from a personal vision, the values exemplified in his or her personal lifestyle, and an ability to articulate that vision and set of values while coaching and mentoring with unbounded passion.[9]

Leaders Use Noncensored Communication

Some leaders censor what they relay to employees, preferring to frame their messages in only positive terms. Censored communication deprives people from taking responsibility for their behavior and from learning, because it denies them knowledge of what is actually happening and why it has to happen. Organizations that value employee growth and development, even during uncertain times such as those requiring downsizing and cost reduction, often set up employee and customer hot lines to answer questions. Sometimes they form focus groups for employees and interested customers. Some organizations also produce brief videocassettes that employees can take home to help answer questions their families and neighbors might have. Managers who want employees to be truthful, open, and candid should role-model the behavior they expect from their employees.

Leaders Use Self Properly

"Too often in the management of change," says Peggy Nazarey, director of nursing, Harbor-UCLA Medical Center, "we focus outside of our 'self' for the answers that make it happen." Many others agree with her observation and advocate that the "instrument of self" is among a transformational leader's most important tools. According to Nazarey:

> The instrument of self has both "hard" and "soft" skills. Hard elements are those skills that are built and developed from a specific body of knowledge, such as organizational theory, systems theory, and

management theory. Soft elements are those personal skills and attributes that are developed from the interaction with the environment of
the individual's inner beliefs, values, and personality. . . . Transformational leaders have unique abilities and styles. However, the successful transformational leader has a mix of both hard and soft skill
elements that are excellently executed at varying degrees depending on
need. Perhaps the one factor that integrates the instrument of self most
is the value and belief that leadership is both a privilege and responsibility. When we take responsibility to lead people and organizations in
a change process, the transformational leader's job is not complete until
all have arrived safely, in the future, carrying the skills they will need
to function there.

Leaders Are Champions for Change, Politicians, and Negotiators

Transformational leaders champion change, innovation, and creativity, rather
than maintain tight control and keep the big picture for the organization
to themselves. Sharon Lee, vice-president of patient care services, St. Luke's
Regional Medical Center, explains her transformational leader role this way:

> I function as a resource, coach, catalyst, and a networker within the
> organization, the community, and beyond. I must be a politician, assess-
> ing the environment and gaining support for change; a negotiator when
> necessary, achieving harmony, community spirit, and mutually agreed-
> upon outcomes; an orchestrator of events and processes; and a master
> at resolving conflicts that are sure to arise in this climate of turbulence
> and uncertainty.

The context of change requires everyone's understanding; boundaries
must be clear and open for honest and heartfelt interaction. Alliances resulting from change often are built on the hopes and dreams of the future, but
also require the realities of consensus, direction, defined processes, and realis-
tic expectations for all involved. Achieving the balance between what is
desired and what can be achieved may require the talents of negotiation
and persuasion to reach consensus.

Leaders Are Stewards

A *steward* is someone who has a sense of ownership and accountability for
the well-being of the organization as a whole system, recognizing the importance of structure and direction and yet allowing freedom of choice for everyone involved. *Stewardship* is a spiritual dimension built on the core of a
personal value system; it inspires commitment and a sense of common
ownership by every stakeholder in the organization. Within the patient-

centered care philosophy a steward maintains a focus on providing the best value for meeting the needs of the patient in the most appropriate care settings.

Leaders Are Contemplatives

A *contemplative* is an individual who is disciplined to set aside time for regular quietness and solitude to examine his or her life, relationships with others, efforts within the organization, and contribution to the community and society at large. In his book *A World Waiting to Be Born,* Peck writes: "Contemplative time is a life style dedicated to maximum awareness. Those who use it desire to become as conscious of reality as they can possibly be."[10] In a 1994 article in *Fortune* magazine, Sherman writes:

> The shift from machine-age bureaucracy to flexible, self-managing teams requires that lots of ordinary managers and workers be psychologically prepared to push the transformation themselves. . . . To the degree that individuals are successful at plumbing their depths, those people should be better off, and the companies that employ them may gain competitive advantage. . . . There's more to us than the sniveling, snarling organism that craves power and approval. The clarity and contentment we seek lies deep inside us all.[11]

Leaders Care for the Soul of Individuals and the Organization

In his book *Soulmates,* Moore regards relationships from the viewpoint of soul; that is, people who work together soulfully are fulfilling their collective destiny.[12] This perspective fosters acceptance of differences among stakeholders as they work together to achieve common goals. It also may allow true tolerance beyond judgments of good or bad, and may recognize pain and failure as sources of deepening commitment to a greater, more altruistic purpose. In an article in *Administrative Radiology Journal,* Paul Ill asserts that leaders who care for the individual soul are passionate. Their work and beliefs are one and the same, putting the needs of others above their own.[13] These leaders empathize with those seeking and providing services, focusing on their dreams and fantasies and establishing intraorganizational collaborative relationships while identifying interventions or solutions for the improvement of services and quality of work life. Dominick Flarey, administrator and COO, Youngstown Osteopathic Hospital, sums it up: "A leader who is faith-filled displays a strong faith in the ability of the people, the organization, and the health care system to change and grow."

Leaders Have Integrity and Respect Colleagues

Transformational leaders "walk the talk" rather than just "talk the talk." This includes relating to others with integrity, trust, respect, sincerity, genuineness, and acceptance. Their integrity provides the foundation for respect from others and is the building block for mutual respect throughout the organization. Annette McBeth, vice-president, Immanuel-St. Joseph's Hospital, says that *integrity* means: "I can be counted on. If I say I will do something, there is assurance that it will happen or an explanation will be provided." Within this context, the term's attributes include feedback and follow-up. Thus, transformational leaders demonstrate their integrity through their actions; they are highly ethical and communicate their message consistently and directly during the change process. If they do not, the results can be disastrous. Thomas Mroczkowski, vice-president/COO, Hackley Hospital, warns: "I believe a single lapse of integrity can destroy the effectiveness of the leader throughout an organization."

Leaders Are Catalysts for Creativity and Innovation

Creativity is needed to generate alternative approaches to problem and issue resolution. If people are uncomfortable with the idea of suggesting alternatives, innovations will not happen. Thus, effective leaders encourage employees to risk being creative. As James Sauer, senior vice-president/director of the Health Care Division, Alexander & Alexander of California, observes: "It is the role of senior management to encourage critical thinking, setting the stage for safe expression of ideas and use of imagination by people to achieve innovations."

Leaders Are Facilitators

The transformational leader's ability to achieve consensus among diverse constituencies is critical to the success of any change process. To arrive at consensus means allowing people the opportunity to work out personal differences, to find strengths and commonalities on which to build, and to learn together how to reach desired goals. Thus, transformational leaders must facilitate the change process, rather than direct it. In addition to listening to the message, leaders must listen to how it is said. The facilitator role requires that the transformational leader possess good communication skills, be objective, and be sensitive to people's needs and concerns.

Leaders Function as Team Members

The ability of the transformational leader to function as a team member, whether on the executive team or a small task force, is critical to innovation and improvement processes. William Manahan, medical director of quality assurance, Immanuel-St. Joseph's Hospital, explains the importance of this characteristic from a physician's perspective:

> To be a team player and co-creator requires the ability to listen, compromise, let go of control, and ask for help. A key attribute for a physician involved in a team process is to believe in the intrinsic worth of each person on the team. Part of the difficulty for physicians to embrace team attributes is that we often are trained in a manner assuring that we will be "captain of the ship." You are the one ultimately responsible for this patient. It is your scalp if something goes wrong. The physician knows who is sued if there is a problem. There are few other care providers who, as part of their professional role, take calls 7 days a week, 24 hours a day, managing the care of a hospitalized patient. The burden of responsibility weighs heavily on the physician leader, and we often easily become excessively controlling. I now tend to give more emphasis on process, appreciating the role of each member of the team, and I am more willing to compromise.

Leaders Practice Personal Learning and Encourage Organizational Learning

Because hospitals are becoming learning organizations, promoting and practicing constant personal learning throughout the hospital is as much the transformational leader's responsibility as it is that of education and human resources personnel. The transformational leader must not only set an example by personal behavior, he or she also must demonstrate a belief in organizational learning and support those who are doing it.

Leaders Are People Centered

People at all levels of the organization need to know that their leadership values what they have to say and how they do their work. One way the transformational leader can accomplish this is by making the effort to converse with people in their work environment. This demonstrates leadership's interest in them as individuals. Also, listening to staff members' ideas and encouraging their input can create positive feelings and promote loyalty to the organization. Sometimes it can have the added benefit of generating staff ideas on how to improve productivity or resolve problems that might otherwise go unaddressed. Additionally, because the transformational leader often must address diverse points of view and facilitate consensus to reach solutions to problems, it is to his or her benefit to develop relationships with people at all levels of the organization. Wayne Frieders, vice-president of human resources, St. Luke's Regional Medical Center, supports this characteristic of transformational leaders:

Meeting customer needs and helping staff do the same by recognizing small and large successes or accomplishments are significant influences on the outcome of care of patients and their families. Leaders must provide resources to bring out the best in people, expect the best, challenge them, and allow them to grow and develop at their pace, even while making some mistakes.

Leaders Use Holistic Approaches

Transformational leaders are holistic in their approach, dealing with the environment, the community, and society at large in a proactive and prospective manner.[14-17] Barbara Donaho found that her role as an executive health care leader included a commitment to building a healthier community, which energized her to become a board member of the Chamber of Commerce, Goodwill Industries, and United Way. She also became actively involved with multiple downtown development and neighborhood coalitions, parish nursing programs, and other social and health related endeavors.

Leaders Empower Others

Another important characteristic of transformational leaders is their willingness to empower employees. If given the tools and mentored toward self-direction, empowered employees will make suggestions for opportunity realization they are capable of achieving. However, although empowerment is a powerful tool, it is not an end in itself. It requires structure, expectations, and constant focus on what is best for patients and their families, the organization, and the community. A team structure expands opportunities for empowerment, because team members draw security, trust, and reinforcement from each other while testing the new environment.

Leaders Recognize That Relationships Are Vital to Restructuring and Transition

Relationship building is key to the success of restructuring in and outside the organization. Skills in collaboration, interdependence, and cocreation are the outgrowths of effective and meaningful relationships.[18] Hammer and Kanter indicate that interinstitutional relationships work best when they are familylike and less rational. Because relationships involve the emotions, trust, values, and experiences of the parties involved, they should not be entered into lightly, especially if sustained change is desired and long-term efficiencies are expected.[19,20] It is important that the organization create a familylike environment for employees. Managers at all levels are responsible for showing employees that they care about them, whether or not the employees stay with the company. In addition to showing that they care, managers also must give employees the tools and training they need to develop their skills and knowledge.[21,22] The result is an institution with self-reliant workers who can thrive and pay attention not only to themselves but also to a greater good (such as the community they serve and society at large).

Change can be intensely personal and people may have to give up something in the process. Recognition of that loss and allowance for a grieving process will bring fears and discomfort to the surface. Sharon Lee cautions that "that trust may be shaken until people understand why the change is occurring and how they will be affected personally and professionally. However, the process of rebuilding trust must be done systematically by the leadership with sensitivity for the individual while achieving an outcome for the whole organization." Annette Compton, director of volunteers, St. Luke's Regional Medical Center, describes how unsettling restructuring can be:

> From the time the restructuring at St. Luke' Regional Medical Center was initiated until outcomes were announced was an anxious period for everyone. Where would I fit seemed to be the most common question? It's hard to think about the organization as a whole and the positive benefits of systems redesign when one's job might be drastically changed. However, it is important to maintain an organizational focus while waiting for the outcome. It is equally important to be given the opportunity to express feelings about the coming changes and to provide input as part of the change process.

However, the employees are not the only ones who are affected by the change process. Leaders, too, may be required to make difficult adjustments. As change occurs, leaders must possess flexibility to change roles and even accept a reduction in title in the new environment. Wayne Frieders explains:

> As a part of St. Luke's Regional Medical Center's organizational restructuring process, my title changed from vice-president of human resources to director of human resources. The medical center is transitioning from [a] traditional structure with a top-down reporting relationship to a service design based on centers/institutes. This change will not markedly alter my ability to influence key decisions, but it does alter how I relate with the executive level and establishes a closer connection with managers and unit-level staff. Although the change in title may seem like a demotion, the responsibilities have not decreased nor has the significance of the role with executive leadership. The challenge of change and uncertainty will result in many employees and managers seeking more assistance from the human resource staff, not less. There will be different challenges and growth opportunities for everyone. I will miss, at times, being a part of the first to know what is going on

in the organization. However, since my influence on human resource decisions is based on my skills and knowledge of sound human resource practices, I'm confident that my expertise will be valued and used more appropriately. As long as people continue to come to me with human resource questions and problems and use my counsel and guidance to help their department or the organization, I will continue to have high job satisfaction. The change, from my perspective, was timely and fits the needs of the medical center and enhanced the role for human resources as integral to the organizational strategic plan.

Leaders Often Are Cantadoras, or Tellers of Stories

Visionary leaders often use stories as tools to break resistant behaviors, build trust, achieve new attitudes, and direct collective energy toward a desired outcome. Stories have a way of penetrating an individual's ego to influence his or her spirit. They allow the mind to be receptive to a message that otherwise might be difficult to receive or understand. Project staff from Harbor-UCLA Medical Center agree: "Once a person is hooked on listening to a story, the essence or meaning of the story can be translated to a real-life situation. Stories add a dimension of fun and intuition while bringing insight and acceptance." Margorie Beyers, executive director, American Organization of Nurse Executives, indicates that "An advantage of telling stories is creating an organizational history—the organizational mythology." Thus, stories are one of the strongest tools for generational learning and can become the foundation of an historic journal for institutional change and the basis of dissemination plans in publications and presentations. Edward Foley, regional vice-president, Hospital Council of Southern California, Center of Health Resources, sums up this characteristic of transformational leaders:

> A true transformational leader is an exceptional person. This leader is someone who, through his or her personal actions, changes people's attitudes, goals, and, ultimately, their own actions. Such a person has to be seen as a believer in what he or she says, not just one who talks a good game. He or she must be seen interacting with events in a consistent, forceful way. Such a person must be understood and accepted by the group. Frequently, such a leader is one who can tell "stories" that bring home, in everyday and in human terms, the reason for changes and beliefs through examples of other people who, in similar situations, have effectively coped with new situations with changes in attitudes, beliefs, and behavior.

• Transformational Leaders on their Roles

Following are perspectives on transformational leader roles as experienced by leaders at different levels and in a variety of organizational settings:

- *Lloyd Smith, CEO, MeritCare Health System:* A transformational leader must have the following characteristics:
  - *Instinct and courage:* A risk-taker to make a leap of faith, not wait for everything to be right; go with instinct to do what you feel is right, despite naysayers, and maintain courage for your convictions.
  - *Patience:* Moving towards one's vision requires patience. When denied immediate gratification or results, vision is so important.
  - *Creativity:* Realize and appreciate creativity of those around you; unleash, foster, encourage creativity, not direct it. This is part of the coaching role, looking at how to channel systems and unleash creativity.
  - *Self-confidence and self-esteem:* One will be second-guessing; need to be able to deal with the setbacks; have confidence that you made the right decision even though there may not always be support to pick you up, and have confidence in your ability to be responsive.
  - *Organizational ability:* Able to see the big picture, but yet identify the components; able to rule out redundancy; there is so much activity at the same time that it is hard not to double up and waste resources.
  - *Timing:* Knowing when to take [the] whole thing and run with it, rather than walk; need to deal with the sensitivity of people who have job worth and self-worth tied up in their job title.
- *Joyce Clifford, nurse executive, Beth Israel Hospital:* The following are essential requirements for leadership:
  - The ability to stay close to the issues, predicting and directing the response of others, helping others to understand the issues and helping them to cope with change appropriately.
  - The ability to manage the boundaries of issues well so that integration replaces turf and territorial practices, and interdisciplinary planning and evaluation is accomplished on behalf of those in need of health services.
  - The ability to demonstrate continued personal and professional growth, understanding that yesterday's leadership may not be tomorrow's need.
  - Leadership is not just a job responsibility for some; leadership is the essence of professionalism and should be considered an essential component of all nurse and other professional roles. True leadership is mutual growth and understanding; it is the willingness to be led, as well as to lead; and, of great importance, [it] is to have enough common sense to know when to do which!
- *Joni Stright, CFO, McCall Memorial Hospital:* Leaders are system thinkers, role models, individuals who set the vision, plan for the future, and create a workplace environment that provides opportunities for others to excel. They have charisma and motivate others to achieve a desired outcome. They influence others and facilitate learning so they are effective contributors. Leaders delight in the contributions of staff and set a tone for learning and achieving through group effort — not individual effort. My basic belief, that serves as my daily guide in my role as chief financial officer,

is that all people desire to do what is right and want to do a good job. My leadership role is to facilitate and support their desire to want to do a good job in the following ways:

— Understand priorities for their particular job/department, and facilitate understanding of the priorities for the organization (the vision), assuring that the two are synergistic.

— Protect them from the "small stuff" that can swallow them when they are trying to focus on big priorities; assisting them to learn how to spend time on important and urgent priorities, as opposed to the urgent and not important.

— Mentor them, passing on anything that will facilitate self-motivation; trust their judgment; and communicate directly in a clear, concise manner, allowing them to express ideas and feelings in order that we agree on what is expected for them and for me.

— Look for the good in everything they do; provide them tools to enhance their ability to handle their own problems and issues.

— Enjoy watching others grow, developing their abilities, and observing their successes — this I believe is truly the greatest reward a leader can receive.

— Be passionate about what I do and proactive, never settling for the status quo unless it is meaningful to the organization.

— Enjoy the fun of work. Life is too short not to enjoy what one does personally and professionally.

• *Brian Schreck, vice-president, St Luke's Regional Medical Center:* I firmly believe staff at all levels should have an understanding of the big picture to facilitate their ability to be enthusiastic and effective contributors. . . .

Current organizational restructuring processes have caused me to rethink the way I lead and manage. I am fortunate to be involved with departments which have systems implications: information services, laboratory, medical imaging, human resources, education, security, building services, risk management and safety, and quality improvement. Using the traditional tenets of directing and controlling would be an impossible method of managing. Leadership is expected to provide direction, facilitate interactions, and remove barriers for managers to do their work at the unit level. These managers have been carefully selected, oriented, and trained. In our new way of working, leaders can best model their role by demonstrating a level of teamwork and synergy that is akin to what is exemplified by a championship athletic team. We must no longer feel that we need to master and control all of the information, nor must we believe that we need to have all the answers to all of the questions. . . . No individual can master [all] the information, skills, and expertise needed to be competitive or even viable in a challenging and competitive environment. New leaders and mangers must be competent in certain areas and rely on the knowledge and skills of colleagues in other areas. I would be foolish to pretend I could question a decision made by nurses relative to clinical practice. This requires that we make good decisions as we hire individuals for manager functions at the unit level: They are the ones who will be accountable for decisions close to their work, not executive leaders. There must be a substantial commitment to orient and train to organizational beliefs, especially to what is expected in terms of specific performance. The result will be better decisions that are made expeditiously, customers are delighted, employees are satisfied because they feel that they had something to do with the success of the organization, and the organization will fulfill its mission in a way that is consistent with its values. The mission and values of the organization should be communicated to all employees so they can live them out in their daily work. As leaders let go of traditional methods of management and shift their role to that of facilitators, coaches, and mentors, they may be rewarded with surplus time that can now be spent with families and friends and non-work-related activities. Having time for outside hospital activities refreshes our spirits and helps us remember why we do what we do and to what important end it is all directed.

- *Brad Brown, vice-president of information systems, Tallahassee Memorial Regional Medical Center:* I see myself now more than ever to be an educator, looking at information as an integral part of what we all do; a visionary, linking the islands of today's data into the information architectures of tomorrow; and an interpreter, explaining what technology can and cannot do. . . .

   My primary function is to be a creator and driver of change . . . reaching beyond the walls of the medical center to clinics and service settings in the community. I am a technology consultant to my peers. I should no longer be considered solely as the titular head of the IS [information services] department, but rather as a resource to address health care system information and management issues. As a leader, I must be prepared to:

  —Facilitate and coach, instead of dictate and supervise
  —Relinquish authority to empowered employees, yet provide them structure
  —Focus on total processes and systems, rather than on discrete tasks taking a holistic approach
  —Manage relationships in the context of the interactive planning process and systems thinking
  —Communicate corporate information strategy to decision makers at all levels of the organization
  —Increase one-on-one, as well as group, conversations and dialogue with staff in my area of responsibility and the areas supported by IS functions
  —Provide internal selling and counseling to employees struggling with change

• Conclusion

Motivation for initiating organizational change can come from examination of the characteristics of successfully transformed organizations that have moved toward patient-centered care delivered through a broad continuum by an interdependent organization seeking value-driven outcomes. Broad characteristics of leaders in this transformation include their ability to creatively model and encourage collaborative staff behavior that is congruent in structure, process, and managerial style throughout the institution. Fostering change in the relationships of the institutions' employees, departments, and divisions is the immediate goal, with the ultimate goal of building interorganizational and intersocietal alliances. Transformational leaders have the need to be proactive, setting their sights on positive pragmatic results (achievements) for the well-being of others and the organization. Such leaders have a passion to lead, incorporating their belief into their work.

References

1. Waterman, R. H., Waterman, J. A., and Collard, B. Toward a career-resilient workforce. *Harvard Business Review* 72(4):87–95, July–Aug. 1994.

2. Stein, M., and Hollwitz, J. *Psyche at Work: Workplace Applications of Jungian Analytical Psychology.* Wilmette, IL: Chiron Publications, 1992.

3. Inguagiato, R. *Organizational Theory: Fundamentals of Medical Management.* Tampa: American College of Physician Executives, 1993.

4. Cummings, T. G., and Worley, C. G. *Organization Development and Change.* 5th Ed. St. Paul: West Publishing Company, 1993.

5. Gibson, J. L., Ivancevich, J. M., and Donnelly, J. H., Jr. *Organizations: Behavior, Structure, Process.* 8th Ed. Burr Ridge, IL: Richard D. Irwin, Inc., 1994.

6. *Bridging the Leadership Gap in Healthcare.* Executive Summary of a National Study Conducted by the Leadership Center of the Healthcare Forum. San Francisco: The Healthcare Forum, 1992.

7. Owen, H. *Leadership Is.* Potomac, MD: Abbott Publishing, 1990.

8. Shortell, S. M., Morrison, E. M., and Friedman, B. *Strategic Choices for America's Hospitals: Managing Change in Turbulent Times.* San Francisco: Jossey-Bass, 1992.

9. Senge, P. M., Roberts, C., Ross, R. B., Smith, B. J., and Kleiner, A. *The Fifth Discipline Fieldbook: Strategies and Tools for Building a Learning Organization.* New York City: Doubleday, 1994.

10. Peck, M. S. *A World Waiting to Be Born: Civility Rediscovered.* New York City: Bantam Books, 1993.

11. Sherman, S. Leaders learn to heed the voice within. *Fortune* 130(4):92–100, Aug. 22, 1994.

12. Moore, T. *Soulmates: Honoring the Mysteries of Love and Relationship.* New York City: HarperCollins, 1994.

13. Ill, P. The passion to lead: transforming accomplishment into achievement. *Administrative Radiology Journal* 13(7):25–28, July 1994.

14. Capra, F. *The Turning Point: Science, Society, and the Rising Culture.* New York City: Bantam Books, 1982.

15. Covey, S. R. *Principle-Centered Leadership.* New York City: Simon & Schuster, 1992.

16. Kaiser, L. R. The visionary manager. In: T. C. Wilson, editor. *Emerging Issues in Health Care 1988.* Estes Park, CO: Estes Park Institute, 1988, pp. 94–104.

17. Wheatley, M. J. *Leadership and the New Science: Learning About Organization from an Orderly Universe.* San Francisco: Berrett-Koehler, 1992.

18. Kanter, M. R. Collaborative advantages: the art of alliances. *Harvard Business Review* 72(4):96–108, July–Aug. 1994.

19. Kanter.

20. Hammer, M., and Champy, J. *Reengineering the Corporation: A Manifesto for Business Revolution.* New York City: HarperCollins, 1993.

21. Waterman, Waterman, and Collard.

22. Whiteside, J. *The Phoenix Agenda.* Essex Junction, VT: Oliver Wright Publications, Inc., 1993.

Part Two

Identifying Opportunities for Change

• Introduction to Part 2

During his best moments, the visionary leader touches the mind of the universe, and initiates a structuring vision that becomes a dynamic grid attracting the elements necessary for its fulfillment. The strategic plan of the hospital should be this type of structuring vision for the future. A good plan is a description of a desired destination and a strategy for getting there. If the board, medical staff and management are caught up in the planning effort, the resulting vision will renew the organization and regenerate the energies of everyone involved.

The Visionary Manager, Leland R. Kaiser.
In: *Emerging Issues in Health Care 1988*

Part 1 set the stage for organizational transformation, examining the current forces that are compelling change and describing the characteristics of organizations and leaders that have negotiated the change process successfully. Now the questions to be addressed are, How do institutions deal with these forces in practical and actual terms? How do they integrate new types of services and practices with organizational improvement? How do they navigate around barriers and road blocks in traditional top-down decision making, department- or discipline-driven needs response? How do they deal with continuing competition with health care colleagues? Although there is no definitive technique, blueprint, or answer, various solutions are emerging from the collective experiences of many organizations and leaders who are considered pioneers in the health care system.[1-6]

The initial step in organizational transformation is clear: Analyze the specific opportunities for change. These opportunities are defined by comparing desired outcomes with current reality through the visioning processes in the three chapters comprising part 2. Chapter 3, Fulfilling Organizational Vision, overviews the why, who, where, how, and results of visioning, and provides insight into how the visioning process can be maintained for ongoing revisioning as the key to continuous value improvement. Chapter 4, Defining Values and Selecting Opportunities, presents details of visioning using the principles of John Lathrop's Value Framework Process, and defines the methods of The Interactive Planning and Management Process as applied by Alan Barstow. As current reality is altered by attaining defined opportunities, the process of revisioning keeps the desired outcome advancing as a target that is continuously moving toward ultimate improvement. Although the transformational process is depicted in discrete steps and stages, in reality all are occurring simultaneously as the process moves through the organization. At some point in this dynamic and ever-changing process, a critical mass of individuals becomes aware of an "Ah ha" experience in which a sense of new meaning flows through the organization, forming a community united by a common destiny. This experience may be termed the "birth of the organizational soul." As described in chapter 5, Making the Change, when soul is recognized and honored, the organization and its leaders know that something remarkable has taken place and often describe the effects in spiritual terms. Leaders move beyond assumptions and practices to form new awarenesses, insights, and sensibilities.

References

1. Ray, M., and Rinzler, M. *The New Paradigm in Business: Emerging Strategies for Leadership and Organizational Change.* New York City: Jeremy P. Tarcher/Perigee Books, 1993.

2. Senge, P. M. *The Fifth Discipline: The Art and Practice of the Learning Organization.* New York City: Doubleday, 1990.

3. Hammer, M., and Champy, J. *Reengineering the Corporation: A Manifesto for Business Revolution.* New York City: HarperCollins, 1993.

4. Lombardi, D. *Progressive Health Care Management Strategies.* Chicago: American Hospital Publishing, 1992.

5. Covey, S. R. *Principle-Centered Leadership.* New York City: Simon & Schuster, 1992.

6. Whiteside, J. *The Phoenix Agenda.* Essex Junction, VT: Oliver Wright Publications, 1993.

Chapter 3

Fulfilling Organizational Vision

Destiny, like the soul, is the true, authentic self. . . . Destiny is simultaneously personal and communal. It is not possible to describe unambiguously the relationship between destinies, but experience shows the general character of these relationships. . . . Our dignity consists in our possession of destinies and is affirmed through fidelity to our destinies.

Against Fate: An Essay on Personal Dignity, Glenn Tinder

To be the leader of an organization in which all the stakeholders are content with its current market share and service delivery would be enviable. However, hard-learned lessons in the history of management tell us that contentment with the status quo can lead to complacency and blind an organization to outside forces that might require it to change. Such was the case a few years ago with the U.S. automotive industry as foreign manufacturers quietly and effectively captured market share with cars that were perceived by the American public to have greater value (high quality and low price). Management and stockholders of giant corporations such as General Motors, Ford, and Chrysler were stunned by the success of their foreign competitors, evidently because the American manufacturers had assumed that their current reality was synonymous with their desired future; that is, their satisfaction with the status quo blinded them to possible opportunities for value improvement. As described in this chapter, the visioning process could have tested the validity of their assumption. Although visioning focuses on the desired outcome, when agreement is reached by all participants, current reality stands out in stark comparison. The differences between the current reality and the desired future are opportunities for improvement.

This chapter describes the visioning process and presents questions that organizational leaders might consider to measure its impact. It also presents a list of principles that serve to guide organizations and their leaders as they fulfill their vision.

• The Visioning Process

The visioning process is the crucible that encourages participants to align themselves and their units or departments with the soul and destiny of the organization, as well as with the community. An organization that is grounded in and guided by its mission and values is fulfilling its deeper purpose, or *destiny* and honoring its true essence, or *soul.* By aligning themselves with that destiny, the organization's stakeholders show they understand the common goals that have been determined by a systematic process of defining and agreeing on the organizational vision. Absolutely critical to appropriate and effective organizational transformation is the initial setting of a vision, participated in and owned by all the stakeholders, including customers and suppliers, both internal and external. Through interaction, ranging from casual conversations to formal group processes, hospital executives and trustees, employees, physicians, and patients and their families alike can agree on a common understanding of the organization's destiny. It is only through such dialogue that the true destiny of the organization can be defined.[1] The stakeholders reach agreement by sharing their understanding of what the organization should be and what it should do for their community. Their common desire to design a system of care that values patient-centeredness, continuity of care across hospital and community service settings, appropriate and efficacious services, collaborative relationships with physicians and businesses, and appropriate utilization of professional and support staff is the most compelling force behind arriving at a vision that is endorsed by everyone.

Building a shared vision provides all members of the health care institution the opportunity to reach the goal of creating an integrated, holistic care delivery system for a healthier community—one that melds social responsibility with the corporate responsibility of business. Such a vision regards the healing and spiritual aspects of the organizational mission and values to be of equal or greater importance than financial performance. When major organizational stakeholders participate in this type of relationship and engage in dialogue, they become cocreators in restoring proper relationships throughout their organization and community.

An organizational vision often starts as the personal goal of the institution's chief executive officer (CEO), and is influenced and strengthened through conversations with and among leadership team members, trustees, employees, physicians, patients and their families, and sometimes business coalitions and other community members. Questions may be raised as to why the hospital could not perform a specific service or whether a service could be performed more efficiently or cost-effectively. Business coalitions may request packaged services or employee health contracts to create health care and cost efficiencies for themselves. Often elements come from new opportunities in health services as perceived by social agencies or community parishes. However and wherever visioning starts, there usually exists a shared sense of wanting to advance the organizational mission and values to improve the health status of the community.

Lloyd Smith, president/CEO, MeritCare Hospital, indicates that initiating a visioning process "sometimes takes a leap of faith to do something different, even when some employees or physicians will not understand or accept it." He adds that compelling forces, both inside and outside the organization, usually will stimulate reflection as to the organization's purpose. Many futuristic and system experts emphasize that visioning should include attentiveness to the intellectual, emotional, social, and spiritual dimension of the organization and the community.

• Results of the Visioning Process

Organizational life dramatically changes after an effective visioning process has occurred. After going through the process, one executive commented: "I feel our people can now speak from their heart about what really matters to them and what they can do to make this organization better for our patients, the community in which we live, and for ourselves." As shared visioning is experienced throughout the organization, the strength, talents, and competencies of both care providers and leadership are recognized and valued. Leaders understand, respect, and value the resources that exist among employees and physicians, and recognize the community expectations of their organization. This generates greater openness and curiosity among staff who normally are quiet.

According to Smith, an institutionwide visioning process was key to giving common direction to the stakeholders at MeritCare Hospital. Called Odyssey 2,000, this vision became the motivational point of focus, both personally and professionally, for the hospital's executive leaders, board of trustee members, physicians, and associates (care providers, managers, and other employees). Smith knew at the outset that "building a shared vision was the right thing to do" for integration of the strategic directions of Odyssey 2,000, which included long-term performance and human resource strategies, quality improvement initiatives, and a patient-centered care delivery system (PCCDS) that integrated services across a continuum of settings. Without the process at the outset, MeritCare Hospital would have had difficulty accomplishing the massive restructuring, work and role redesign, and reduction in operational and clinical inefficiencies that it did.

Some executives confessed that they were unconvinced that agreeing on a shared vision or understanding organizational destiny was necessary to determining strategic direction. It was only later, when they attempted cost reduction and other survival measures to ensure the hospital's viability in an increasingly competitive marketplace and its smooth operation within an increasingly chaotic internal environment, that they recognized the compelling need to refocus staff and redefine work. They now enthusiastically agree that this is best accomplished through an organizationwide visioning process to align personal and professional goals with those of the organization.

Although financial performance and market share may influence organizational vision, they are not its primary driving force. A hospital administrator from St. Mary's Health Services in Grand Rapids, Michigan, indicates that in that community, local business coalitions are taking the lead for managed care initiatives and pushing hospitals to define services in a manner that sets them apart from other institutions within the geographic area. He refers to this phenomenon as *collaborative competition,* meaning that hospitals are considering integrated care delivery networks to create cost efficiencies even while recognizing and honoring individual differences. Pressure from the business community has stimulated redefinition of the hospital's vision based on the uniqueness of its organizational mission and values. Using the principles of interactive planning and systems thinking, the hospital expanded its vision to encompass its mission's purpose — to provide physical and spiritual healing through collaborative competition.

• Guiding Principles for Leaders and Organizations Fulfilling Their Shared Vision

As organizations articulate, build, and share their vision, their stakeholders embrace different, more creative patterns of thought and behavior, and new models, principles, and archetypes of performance are eagerly explored and tested. The models, policies, and principles that guided them in the past become outmoded and inefficient. Maintaining the status quo or undergoing incremental change is plausible only if it is consistent with the organization's mission and values and if, ultimately, it encourages growth that is aligned with organizational destiny. Once the vision is endorsed throughout the organization, leaders facilitate its actualization to improve performance and increase value. They no longer are guided by hierarchial ideologies and polices of liberal or conservative organizational politics. In *The Soul of Politics,* Jim Wallis writes: ". . . liberalism is unable to demonstrate the kind of values that undergird any serious transformation, and conservatism denies the reality of structural injustice and social oppression."[2] Transformational organizations expect all stakeholders to take personal responsibility for change. They promote personal development for everyone and return to the humanistic values of dignity, trust, respect, and compassion while considering the social concerns of the organization and the community it serves. They encourage strategic thinking and collaborative alliances based on an organizational structure within which people create collaboratively. Leaders do not control and direct; rather, they coordinate a self-organizing, self-renewing, and self-transcending system. They ensure that the resources and means necessary are available to achieve the value desired for patients, their families, the community, and society.

The principles guiding leaders as they fulfill organizational destiny are aggregated and come from a review of current organizational literature, the experience of the SHNP projects, and comments from the contributors to this book.[3-8] These principles include:

- Create a substantive, shared vision known to everyone at all levels of the organization and recognized by members of the community.
- Commit to a patient-centeredness philosophy for patient care delivery.
- Endorse a continuity of care system that provides and integrates consistent, appropriate, and efficacious care across service settings.
- Ensure high-quality and responsive service experiences for customers that are equally satisfying and efficient for those both providing and receiving them.
- Formulate connections and strengthen relationships among all managers, care providers, patients and their families, and the community.
- Encourage the early, active involvement of executive management, the board of trustees, and physicians.
- Institute interactive planning, system thinking, quality (value) improvement, learning organization, and other creative and imaginative processes among individuals from many different levels and departments within and outside the institution and with patients and their families.
- Move from individual accountability to group or team accountability, creating a "teamness" that can progress to interdependence and cocreation.
- Empower employees, patients, and families, recognizing them as a source of knowledge and creativity by supporting their involvement in decision-making processes at the level closest to the patient.
- Implement developmental opportunities early in the change process for all levels of management, physicians, trustees, and care providers by facilitating their ability to contribute in a meaningful manner to organizational, departmental, and unit goals.
- Involve operational support functions such as human resources, pastoral care, information systems, financial systems, management engineering, environmental services, and others.
- Establish valid and effective communication methods that cross organizational boundaries.
- Develop mechanisms for collecting, analyzing, trending, and managing information used to assess and evaluate interventions, and for reporting the information in a manner that is understandable by executive leaders, managers, and unit staff.
- Address the organization's future economic, legal, and competitive struggles as opportunities for partnership and cocreation among employees,

physicians, payers, policymakers, unions, and community social and health services.

- Form linkages with community members such as businesses, parishes, social service agencies, social clubs, and others who have an investment in creating a healthier community.
- Plan for an effective health care work force by forming linkages with educational institutions at the primary, secondary, community college, and university levels.

• Key Elements in the Shift to New Ways of Thinking and Behaving

Key to the process of shifting the organization to new ways of thinking and behaving while operationalizing the principles listed in the preceding section is the ability of its leaders to build connective and interdependent relationships. Following are descriptions of the most important ingredients in the relationship-building process. Transformation leaders must:

- Understand themselves
- Provide open and effective communication systems
- Model personal values
- Achieve a sense of harmony
- Use their imagination

Leaders Understand Themselves

Transformational leaders must learn to understand their personal strengths and the areas in which they need to grow. As one executive puts it: "It takes as much courage to understand one's own response to change as it does to initiate the change process. . . . It is somehow easier to help someone else with resistance, than deal with my own, especially acknowledging that my own resistance affects the whole process." It was with the help of a trusted colleague that another executive came to identify what she wanted for the organization and what stood in her way from reaching her desired goal of becoming a transformational leader. She learned that, as the CEO, she was fearful of not being the expert. She felt she had to have answers and implement the right strategies to posture her organization as a significant service provider in the community. She said: "The board of trustee members, physicians, and employees look to me for direction. What if I do not know the right way; what if I make a mistake?" Once she understood her own resistance and worked through relationship-building processes with board members, senior managers, physicians, other managers, and unit staff throughout the institution, she became excited about involving others. She publicly recognized the competencies and talents of people she had not acknowledged previously, realizing the importance of allowing others to feel a part of the greater purpose of the organization and using one of the learning organization principles promoted by Peter Senge that "people are more intelligent together than they are apart."[9,10] With this change in perspective came a new organizational energy: Everyone was expanding his or her capacity to contribute; people were treating each other as colleagues, using imagination, taking risks, and assessing results. The organization developed a "teamness" that had not existed previously. Developing this teamness provides the basis for transformational leaders to shift an organization from individual accountability to team accountably. Barbara Donaho, SHNP director, emphasizes that team accountably, especially for an institution that has institutionalized a PCCDS, fosters a continuity of care across service settings. This patient-centered care is responsive to patient needs. It shifts the value to what patients and their families need for a high-quality health care outcome from what the department or discipline needs to provide the service.[11,12] In this system, care is given the patient by the appropriate care provider in the appropriate care setting. Meeting the needs of patients and their families may involve multiple disciplines from inpatient and outpatient areas. It is through planning and managing patient care collaboratively that true value results.

Leaders Provide Open and Effective Communication Systems

Open and effective communication systems, particularly those that support dialogue, are essential to building team accountability. In their works, Senge, Bohm, Schein, and Isaacs define *dialogue* as sustained collective inquiry into the processes, assumptions, and certainties that compose everyday experiences.[13-16] Dialogue is at the foundation of interactive processes, systems thinking, and the hospital's transformation to a learning organization. It facilitates the team or group's ability to build common ground and mutual trust, providing a safe environment in which to speak openly and honestly.[17] Leaders at Abbott-Northwestern Hospital, in Minneapolis, indicate that learning to use effective communication techniques institutionwide took much more time than they had anticipated. However, the value added to the hospital greatly outweighed the cost of development. Without effective communication, the successes they have achieved through *innovation,* their theme for institutional integration and improvement, would not have been possible. Innovation is built on the shared vision that "patients are the reason we exist and people are the reason we excel." It is a model for redesign and change set within a framework of systems thinking, interactive planning, reengineering, and the principles of a learning organization.[18] Its goals are to increase patient and family satisfaction; increase operational efficiency and effectiveness; provide more meaningful work within the institution; and increase clinical effectiveness and reduce costs.

Leaders Model Personal Values

Trust, mutual respect, hospitality, acceptance, and compassion are among the values exemplified by people working in an organization that is committed to the principles of transformation through the visioning process using community building and dialogue. Transformational leaders can set the example for these values through their personal attitudes and behaviors. If they do not, employees are less likely to become invested in the organization's vision and destiny. As Joe Caroselli, CEO, Idaho Elk's Rehabilitation Hospital, in Boise, Idaho, states: "Until trust and mutual respect are experienced by the employees, they have difficulty investing and taking ownership beyond their own individual interests. . . . The "what is in it for me" phenomenon pervades if trust is lacking."

However, he also points out that modeling these values is not just important for employees within the organization. Along with St. Luke's Regional Medical Center; four rural hospitals (Holy Rosary Medical Center in Ontario, Oregon; McCall Memorial Hospital in McCall, Idaho; Walter Knox Memorial Hospital in Emmett, Idaho; and Wood River Medical Center in Hailey and Sun Valley, Idaho); and Boise State University, Elk's Rehabilitation Hospital is a member of an intra-agency rural system of care delivery called The Rural Connections: Linking for Healthier Communities whose purpose is to strengthen overall regional health care. Caroselli says that leadership values are equally important in building relationships between the member hospitals of The Rural Connection. "Until we [the leadership from each of the six member hospitals] had trust and respect for each other, we were not able to develop and implement the consortium goal of designing an integrated service for cardiac patients and eventually other patient groups."

Leaders Achieve a Sense of Harmony

Edward Foley, regional vice-president, Hospital Council of Southern California, talks of the transformational leader's responsibility to achieve harmony while shifting from an old way of working to a new vision. He says:

> A major job of the leader is to achieve harmony as people work together to define their clear goal. In meetings or visits to work sites, the leader talks about the organization's vision in terms relevant to each audience. This accomplishes at least two things: (1) The vision is again and again being expressed in real and human terms; and (2) employees see themselves as contributors to the enterprise and its vision because of the close interaction with the leader.

Foley was one of the initial cocreators of the vision for the Harbor-UCLA Medical Center, Torrance, California, entitled A Community of Patient

Care Leaders. The program's design team was a partnership model including executive leaders, managers, staff, physicians, and patients. As partners, they are working to develop new strategies to achieve high-quality patient care, high-quality work life, and organizational effectiveness. The core concept is based on the beliefs that the future requires a shared sense of community and that everyone is a leader.

Leaders Use Their Imagination

The executive leaders of Providence Portland Medical Center in Portland, Oregon, share their belief that imagination is another key ingredient for transformational leaders trying to shift an organization from old paradigms to new guiding principles. Along with applying the work of Senge and Ackoff, the leaders of the Medical Center are using some of Morgan's teachings on "imaginization." *Imaginization* is about improving our ability to see how something works, developing new ways of thinking, and reimaging ourselves and what we do through the use of metaphors, group exercises, and simulations to create insights and new or different images of how something can be done.[19] Morgan's principles include using fun, humor, and hard work to move from top-down, hierarchical management to an open, interactive, and responsive environment. The Medical Center created a visual aid from a child's busy box (a plastic toy with multicolored levers and gears) to describe how relationships between departments affect a patient care delivery system. When the gears are connected and the crank is moving in the correct direction, the system works smoothly; however, if the crank is turned in the wrong direction, the gears lock and the system stops. Each colored wheel represents a different discipline and the crank represents the patient. The model demonstrates the internally cohesive relationships necessary to meet the patient's need for service.

• Impact of the Visioning Process

Organizations differ significantly in how they use visioning and how deeply they are penetrated by the process. Comparisons of such organizations focus on the relationships existing among hospital leadership team members and on the verbal and nonverbal behaviors of managers and staff from different disciplines and levels of an institution. To assess the impact of the visioning process on any organization, the organization's leadership needs to ask itself certain key questions, including:

- Are senior-level leaders working as a team toward a unified goal, or are they individuals espousing a personal or departmental goal?
- Are unit-level managers and staff able to articulate the meaning of their work in relation to the organization's vision, mission, and values?

- Is there a spirit of willingness, harmony, and satisfaction between all levels of managers and staff, and with physicians?
- Are managers tied to traditions or trapped in organizational politics?
- How are strategic decisions made? Is the process top down or interactive? Are multiple disciplines included from all levels?
- What is the value placed on individuals? Are they viewed as contributors bringing knowledge, talent, and creativity to the hospital's work, or are they seen as means to the end?
- What value does the hospital place on the community? Are the community's needs addressed in the hospital's strategic plan?

The answers to these questions should reveal two possible organizational scenarios: those organizations that took time to build a shared vision throughout the institution early in the change process, and those that struggled to operationalize their vision and then build a shared vision late in the change process.

• Health Care Leaders on the Importance of Visioning

Following are the observations of three transformation leaders on the importance of personal and organizational visioning:

Edward Foley, regional vice-president, Hospital Council of Southern California: The delivery of health care in America is in the middle of a revolution. Market forces and governmental action are changing and ultimately will improve health care in America. This revolution will contribute to the growing understanding that medical/hospital care is not the secret to good health in America; rather, it is lifestyle, environment, and many other things. Health insurance will be undertaken by organizations (private or governmental) that will be incentivized to maintain healthy people in their membership. This focus on healthy lives, rather than on the number of high-tech procedures, will change the careers of medical and hospital personnel everywhere, and the system will be better. The way to prepare people to cope with and achieve success through the coming change is to help them see and understand the causes of these changes, the difficulties and challenges these changes present to their organizations, and the need to work together with a clear focus on a vision of the future to achieve success.

Dominick Flarey, administrator/CEO, Youngstown Osteopathic Hospital and executive consultant, Coopers & Lybrand Consulting: The major compelling reason to change how health care services are delivered is the patient. The patient is the foundational element of our business and is the reason health care systems exist. For too long, health care executives have been caught up in a world of competition, one that is market driven to meet the needs of the organization. As such, we have focused our efforts on creating complexities, encouraging destructive organizational politics, developing new services for the sake of revenue gains—all without a core focus on the patient and on caring. For this reason, we are a system that is broken and in desperate need of transformation.

We are quick to place blame on the government for all of the inadequacies in our system. True, such external forces do share in the responsibility for our current dilemma in health care. I believe, however, that the forces internal to our organizations are the major cause of a health care system in trouble. We have created the chaos, or the disease, and only we can fix it.

The prescription for a diseased system is transformation. Transformation simply [the] means to make something new, something better. The organization, the delivery of care, and the people of the organization must all be transformed. I believe that all three of these elements can be transformed together. All interact synergistically to create a system of health care services. Some proposed interventions for a systems integration include:

- *Visionary leadership:* This is imperative for transformation. Leaders must paint a vision for the future and aggressively sell that vision to everyone in the organization. . . .
- *Integration:* True transformation can never be realized unless there is integration. All walls and barriers of the system must be torn down. The concept of departments must be sacrificed for newer and better models leading to organizational integration. Everyone works in partnerships to provide health care services.
- *Redesigned delivery systems:* New, more efficient and effective delivery systems must be designed. Such systems must be primarily focused on the integration of all services of the organization. The core feature of the system is the patient, and redesign must be strategically focused around patients and their needs.
- *A passion for caring:* A strong mission and philosophy of caring must be established and lived out constantly within the organization. The reason our health care system is broken is that we have lost sight of our mission for caring. If everyone in the organization really understood, at a basic feeling level, what our business is, and how significantly we impact each others' lives, then we all would be committed to the integrated delivery of service. Outcomes of a system that cares are efficacious, efficient, and effective. A caring system would have few, if any, quality or productivity concerns.

Winnie Hageman, principal, The Umbdenstock-Hageman Partnership: Commitment by the leadership of the organization is the key to success. While the cornerstone of that leadership is the chief executive officer, the support and commitment of the board of trustees is absolutely critical. The

Board may not be intimately involved in the visioning process, but their commitment to its success can help sustain it.

• Conclusion

As we transform our health care to the systems of the future, the first steps are to test current organizational assumptions and to challenge traditions by creating a vision that pushes beyond the boundaries of departments and disciplines and considers the destiny of the organization in the setting of community need. Leaders of these organizations seek opportunities, not only for themselves but for all stakeholders, to overcome old ideas and notions and to allow all to embrace a vision that supports continuously improved value. Such leaders can relay on a number of guiding principles that others have defined in attempting to fulfill visions for their organizations.

References

1. Isaacs, W. N. *Taking Flight: Dialogue, Collective Thinking, and Organizational Learning. Dia•Logos.* Cambridge, MA: Organizational Learning Center at Massachusetts Institute of Technology, 1994, pp. 24–39.

2. Wallis, J. *The Soul of Politics.* Maryknoll, NY: The New Press and Orbis Books, 1994.

3. Aiken, L., and Fagin, C. *Charting Nursing's Agenda for the 1990s.* Philadelphia: J. B. Lippincott Co., 1992.

4. Charns, M. P., and Smith Tewksbury, L. J. *Collaborative Management in Health Care: Implementing the Integrative Organization.* San Francisco: Jossey-Bass, 1993.

5. Flarey, D. L. *Redesigning Nursing Care Delivery.* Philadelphia: J. B. Lippincott Co., 1994.

6. Marszalek-Gaucher, E., and Coffey, R. *Transforming Healthcare Organizations, How to Achieve and Sustain Organizational Excellence.* San Francisco: Jossey-Bass, 1990.

7. Shortell, S. M., Morrison, E. M., and Friedman, B. *Strategic Choices for America's Hospitals: Managing Change in Turbulent Times.* San Francisco: Jossey-Bass, 1992.

8. Rovin, S., and Ginsberg, L. *Managing Hospitals: Lessons from the Johnson & Johnson-Wharton Fellows Program in Management for Nurses.* San Francisco: Jossey-Bass, 1991.

9. Senge, P. M., Roberts, C., Ross, R. B., Smith, B. J., and Kleiner, A. *The Fifth Discipline Fieldbook: Strategies and Tools for Building a Learning Organization.* New York City: Doubleday, 1994.

10. Senge, P. M. *The Fifth Discipline: The Art and Practice of the Learning Organization.* New York City: Doubleday, 1990.

11. Kohles, M. K., and Donaho, B. A. Twenty-grantees seek transformation: from discipline-driven compartmentalized entities to patient-driven, unified care systems. *Strategies for Health Care Excellence* 5(11):1–12, Nov. 1992.

12. National Program Office. *Strengthening Hospital Nursing: A Program to Improve Patient Care, Gaining Momentum: A Progress Report.* St. Petersburg, FL: Robert Wood Johnson Foundation and Pew Charitable Trusts, 1992.

13. Senge and others.

14. Bohm, D. *On Dialogue.* Ojai, CA: David Bohm Seminars, 1990.

15. Senge.

16. Schein, E. H. *On Dialogue, Culture, and Organizational Learning. Dia•Logos.* Cambridge, MA: Institute for Generative Learning and Collaborative Social Change, Inc., 1994, pp. 40–51.

17. Isaacs.

18. National Program Office. *Strengthening Hospital Nursing: A Program to Improve Patient Care National Meeting Brochure and Meeting Resource Notebook.* St. Petersburg, FL: Robert Wood Johnson Foundation and Pew Charitable Trusts, Fall 1994.

19. Morgan, G. *Imaginization: The Art of Creative Management.* Newbury Park, CA: Sage Publications, 1993.

Chapter 4

Defining Values and Selecting Opportunities

The process (of consensus) requires the members to be emotionally present and engaged, frank in a loving, mutually respectful manner, sensitive to each other; to be selfless, dispassionate, and capable of emptying themselves, and possessing a paradoxical awareness of the preciousness of both people and time.

A World Waiting to Be Born: Civility Rediscovered, M. Scott Peck

Two methods for realizing shared vision and managing interactions throughout the organization in order to achieve agreed-upon desired outcomes have proved successful. One method, developed by John Lathrop from Strategic Insights, Los Altos, California, is the Value Framework Process. This is a specific example of how organizational values can be defined, articulated, and communicated. Through this process, the organization can establish a values hierarchy that begins with the mission statement and embraces unit-level values. The second method is the interactive planning and management process, which was influenced by the work of Russell Ackoff and applied by Alan Barstow of Barstow & Associates, Philadelphia. This process involves realization of an ideal design to achieve desired outcomes.

This chapter explores both of these processes and explains how health care organizations and systems can use them to achieve their desired outcomes. The discussion of the value framework process was written by John Lathrop and the discussion on the interactive planning and management process was written by Alan Barstow.

• The Value Framework Process

The value framework process is based on a specialty of management science called *multiattribute utility decision analysis.* However, it is not a numbers or statistics process; rather, it lies at the subjective judgment end of management science. The process is a structured way to ask the right questions of people at all levels of the organization so that values and objectives can be defined in unambiguous, usable ways. Most of the activity consists of meetings of panels of people across the different levels, departments, and units that make up the organization. In the meetings, panelists discuss questions designed to establish their basic values; show how their values interrelate; examine trade-offs between conflicting values; view how performance at each level, department, and unit affects the performance of the organization as a system for maximizing those values; and reveal how performance in relation to those values can be measured. Many questions are difficult to answer because they force people to confront and reveal their value system very clearly. The most challenging questions are *value dilemma questions* (VDQs), which are designed to confront and explicate often painful value trade-offs involving basic issues such as cost control versus adequacy of care. VDQs force development of basic management concepts, such as improving quality of care for the patient while applying cost control constraints. An example of a VDQ for a manager of ancillary service clinics might be: "You are authorized to add one FTE, either in the pain clinic or in outreach prenatal care. All additional aspects (clinic budget, salary, and so forth) are equal. Which do we hire?" The respondent has to make assumptions about the effectiveness of that staff position in reducing pain or improving prenatal care.

The goal of the value framework process is to focus the institution's management and culture on its mission. It does this by discovering and articulating institutional values in a form that is useful for communicating those values and making decisions based on them.

The process operates at an unusual level of analysis, between the two typical management approaches to analyzing an organization's values — quantitative methods and prose methods:

1. *Quantitative methods:* With quantitative methods, "objective" data (or whatever numerical data happen to be available) are collected and fed into economic or management models. Quantitative method analyses relate all decisions to economic value or a similar narrow concept of efficiency. Although in an abstract sense, the recommendations of those models are correct:
   - Data requirements are often burdensome, usually involving TQM-like indices that involve great effort simply to collect the data.
   - The underlying philosophy can be disempowering; that is, people are characterized as simply a means to the end of maximizing financial or other numerical indexes.
2. *Prose methods:* Prose methods help articulate values in natural language avoiding the problems of quantitative methods. They are effective for

determining bases of a value system, but typically end products are "motherhood statements" that are:

- Not specific enough to establish a genuine sense of shared vision, value, or culture
- Not specific enough to provide substantial guidance for decisions
- Used as too-general rationales for what the decision maker would do anyway

Because the value framework process operates in the productive middle ground between quantitative and prose methods, it has several benefits. For example:

- The process is based on formally correct quantitative methods but is not limited to numerical measures.
- When direct numerical measures are not available for a particular value or goal, the process represents values with subjective measures of effectiveness or impact and, although subjective, they have quantitative content.
- The process quantifies performance and decision outcomes in terms directly useful for strategic planning and decision guidance at all levels.
- Most broadly, the process addresses human values and concerns on their own merit apart from implications for economic or efficiency-based bottom line.

On one hand, the value framework process is top-down because its focus is on the organization's primary objective—for example, effective community health care—and relates everything else to that. However, it also is a bottom-up process because it reaches up to and consults all levels of the system. Questions are asked at all levels of the organization and the answers are used to define the value framework from the lowest level to the highest. This top-down, bottom-up inclusiveness is especially suited to the primary objective of effective community health care because that includes preventive strategies to keep the community member from consuming health care resources. This demands all levels to relate to one objective (top-down), because different and sometimes nonobvious actions may be called for from different levels. At the same time, many of those nonobvious actions will be less obvious to upper management than to other levels, so it is important that all levels of management be consulted for ideas (bottom-up).

An Overview

Although the value framework process is very flexible and can be attuned to the needs of a particular situation, it generally follows six steps. These are:

1. *Step 1: Values Inventory:* Survey and record existing value statements and documentation of value issues and conflicts, as found in organizational documents, including the following:
   - Existing value, vision, and mission statements; current organization charts; reporting relationships
   - Financial statements; current status of strategic planning and projected strategic planning needs
   - Employee and public relations literature; any value-related literature intended for external parties (patients, providers, suppliers or service area)
2. *Step 2: Interview Round 1, Value Elicitation:* Elicit organizational and personal values through a highly structured process (such as nominal group technique or the Delphi process[1]) of asking VDQs, starting with planning staff and working up to senior executives and all other levels of the organization. (Example VDQs are provided later in this chapter.) Optimal group size is between 6 and 10 people; for more than 10, use groups of representatives. The work groups remain intact throughout the process.
3. *Step 3: Value Analysis, Round 1:* Combine all the findings from steps 1 and 2 into:
   - A values hierarchy linking the value relationships of all levels of the organization (A values hierarchy [discussed later in this chapter] is a process that can be used by organizations to prioritize what is important to them, for example, their organizational values)
   - For each level, a mission statement and a set of decision guidance statements specifying targeted performance measures and desirable interrelationships with other levels
4. *Step 4: Interview Round 2, Value Elicitation:* Revisit the groups used in step 2 at an off-site retreat. At each retreat, present the results of step 3 for discussion/correction/feedback/approval.
5. *Step 5: Value Analysis, Round 2:* Incorporate the inputs from step 4 into the value analysis products listed in step 3.
6. *Step 6: Value Implementation/Dissemination:* Revisit the same work groups in an off-site retreat format to do the following:
   - Present the results.
   - Train all participants in the appropriate use of the results, especially for strategic planning, decision guidance, and interrelationships with other organizational departments and levels.
   - Develop action plans as necessary, including specification of milestones and follow-up meetings to check progress, and apply midcourse corrections.

The value framework process results in a number of products, including:

- One or more graphic images called values hierarchies.
- A set of mission statements/value statements/statements of purpose that define the goals and objectives of each level and department of the organization in clear, unambiguous terms that cohesively unite.
- A set of performance measures or indices, some numerically based and some based on subjective prose scales, so that every decision maker at every level has clear guidance and yet the freedom to make decisions that utilize his or her information and expertise. Decisions will be made that are efficient and cost-effective, yet tie together into a cohesive whole.

The performance measures are actual scales (though they may be subjective prose scales) where each point on the scale is a two-sentence description of that level of performance. They are structured in two different ways: the *values orientation,* gathered and displayed with one set of performance measures for each element of the values hierarchy; and the *organizational orientation,* a set of performance measures for each level and department in the organization.

Elements of the Value Framework Process

Figure 4-1 shows the interrelated elements of the value framework process. The numbers correspond to the order in which the elements are described. Thus, the basic process—discover, articulate, and understand values—is the first element (1). It results in five operational features (the five Cs): communication (internal), consistency, clarity, coherence, and communication (external), which in turn result in three cultural features. Values are encoded in a framework that allows effective internal communication of values, goals, and decision guidance (2). Effective internal communication produces consistent decisions (3) and clarity of purpose (4) in organizational behaviors that combine to result in a coherent organization (5). The values framework also provides a basis for communication of important values messages to external communities (6) (patients, providers, suppliers, and the service area). The coherence of the organization, clarity of purpose, and the value framework itself combine to develop a shared vision (7) of the organization held by all members. The shared vision, the coherence of the organization, and the value framework lead to shared leadership (8); that is, a new management culture where decisions are delegated through a process that utilizes values information elicited from all levels of the organization. Following is a breakdown of the features that comprise the value framework.

Feature 1: Discover, Articulate, and Understand Values

The value framework process discovers and articulates the values of the organization in a form useful for communicating and making decisions based

Figure 4-1.   Nine Interlinked Concepts of the Value Framework Process

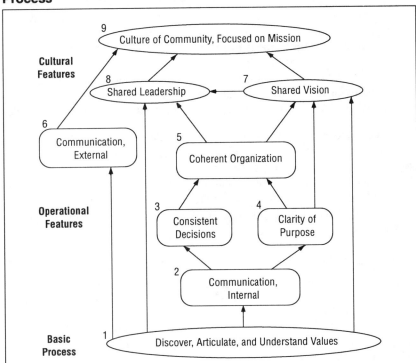

on them. The value framework that results is both a description of those values in a hierarchical structure and a set of performance measures for implementing them. All parties agree on the general aspects of the value framework. That agreement may entail lengthy discussion with deferral of specific details to individual decision makers.

Agreement is neither expected nor sought on a more detailed aspect of the value framework: value trade-offs, or the relative weight given to different values. Trade-offs are elicited using the value dilemma questions mentioned earlier. VDQs may be asked at any of several levels. For example, at the managerial level, a VDQ might be: "You can add one FTE [full-time equivalent] in either pain management/pain management training or outreach prenatal care. Assuming that everything else (remaining budgets, other aspects of health effectiveness, and so on) remains the same, which would you choose?" (The question assumes that adding staff in either of those positions would make sense, be within the appropriate mandate of the hospital, and so on.) Note how the answer to this question reveals a particular value trade-off between different objectives. Although this question is relatively easy to ask, an answer does not reveal value trade-offs "cleanly," because the respondent has to make some assumptions about the effectiveness of the FTE position in reducing pain or improving prenatal care. For that reason, in some cases it is better to ask VDQs at the effects level. The same VDQ asked at the care delivery or unit level would be: "You can reduce pain duration for a given intensity of service of health care by an amount equivalent to 1,000 patient days per year reduced from a "high" to a "medium" index [with "high" and "medium" indices thoroughly defined]; or you can improve prenatal care by an amount equivalent to reducing the number of low-birth-weight babies by 10 per year. Everything else (remaining budgets, other aspects of health effectiveness, and so on) remains the same. Which would you choose?"

With any VDQ, the choice is hypothetical. The particular choice may or may not actually come up in hospital management decisions. However, the value framework process will provide guidance for the choices that *are* made, and that guidance will be *consistent with* the value trade-offs revealed in answers to VDQs.

The value framework process is designed to forge consensus on the general aspects of the value framework, not by forcing people to agree on a particular set of words but by adjusting the level of detail until all parties agree. The result is a common language for understanding the values of the organization/ health care system. This common language is the basis for the other eight elements, five of which are operational and three of which are cultural.

Feature 2: Communication, Internal

Effective communication depends on the concreteness of information. The value framework provides clear interpretations of goals and objectives in terms of performance measures that guide decision making at all levels. Common language developed by the process enables values to be communicated vertically and horizontally throughout all units of the organization in three directions:

- *Top-down:* These are overall goals and values communicated from top executives down to unit teams.
- *Bottom-up:* Unit teams communicate to higher-level decision makers ways to implement those goals and values that apply to more specific situations. Unit-level staff have the most information and knowledge about their tasks, and unit-level staff and lower-level management know more than upper management about how organizational values interface with the demands of operations. Bottom-up communication is key to building a shared vision.

- *Across:* These are goals and values communication from department to department, so that all departments understand each other's goals and objectives.

Internal values communication transmits information related not only to values but also to decision guidance. *Values information* refers to statements or measures describing the values of the organization. *Decision guidance information* refers to prose or quantitative instructions for decision makers. These two types of information are inextricably linked. Values information has no meaning unless it is related to decision guidance, and decision guidance has no consistent basis unless it is rooted in values information. Internal communication is a necessary part of generating information needed to achieve values that are meaningful to everyone.

Feature 3: Consistent Decisions

Internal values communication enables decisions in all parts of the organization to be made consistently. Performance measures provide explicit guidance for decisions at all levels and serve as definitions of values in operational terms. As a result, lower-level (unit) decision makers have clear guidance on how to make decisions; that is, how to make decisions that will maximize performance measures. How they do that is up to them, but what to maximize is defined. For example, unit staff may be asked to decrease labor costs, rather than automatically reduce FTEs, they may change the staff skill mix. By changing the staff skill mix they may actually increase FTEs to achieve the cost savings. (Skill mix refers to the professional staff and support staff ratio.) Performance measures allow decisions to be delegated for efficiency, but with the assurance they will be made consistent with defined goals and objectives.

Feature 4: Clarity of Purpose

Internal communication of values also achieves clarity of purpose, which enables units to cooperate in identifying solutions. Focusing on organizational values and performance measures helps develop creative solutions to particular problems, such as teaching family members how to provide care, showing the need for more volunteer services, or creating new preventive care strategies.

Feature 5: Coherent Organization

Consistency and clarity enable the organization to act coherently, meaning that all parts, guided by decentralized decision making, can act efficiently and effectively in support of the overall organizational mission. Coherence can be viewed from three perspectives:

1. *Communication of values and goals as guidance for integration:* As a basis for collaboration and integration, the value framework process provides a foundation for communicating values and goals between the levels of an organization (vertical integration) and between departments and units at the same level (horizontal integration).
2. *Increased understanding of other decision makers:* Within the value framework, everybody knows what each decision maker is trying to do (achieve high performance as measured by explicit performance measures). Decisions that are consistent and clear enable the organization to be a coherent system focused on its primary mission.
3. *Increased understanding by internal customers:* All unit-level staff members understand their role in the overall organizational mission and its importance. They know who in the institution is their customer.

Feature 6: Communication, External

The value framework process provides a basis for describing the organizational mission and values to external communities: patients, providers, suppliers, and the service area. It enables building a values-based image of the organization in terms relevant to the concerns of its external communities. Using the value framework, the organization can present itself to those communities as cohesive, guided by explicit unambiguous values, and focused on its overall mission.

Feature 7: Shared Vision

Because all levels of the organization are involved in values discovery and articulation, the process enfranchises the entire work force and contributes to an esprit de corps. Guided dialogue involving everyone working on a joint product (the value framework) and focusing on values and concerns rather than positions builds mutual empathy, trust, and respect among decision makers and all members of the organization. The result is development of a shared vision. Employees at all levels see that they are consulted and that their answers will become part of how the institution is managed. As the value framework process proceeds, unit-level staff see that the answers to their questions are reflected in the process itself, in terms of performance measures and the values hierarchy. The net effect is that the employees "own the vision." They feel responsible for improving services because they are part of the process that defines what those services are and how they can be improved, and they feel recognized for their contributions.

Feature 8: Shared Leadership

The value framework enables more effective delegation of decisions. Because values are shared by and defined at all levels of the organization, management by values is management by shared leadership. The value framework process converts an authoritarian–hierarchical management style into shared leadership in two ways:

1. *Multilevel input into the value framework process:* Management staff at all levels, including unit staff members, are consulted to establish the values hierarchy and performance measures.
2. *Multilevel decision making:* Decision making is delegated clearly and completely, because higher levels of management feel comfortable with delegation under the structure of the values hierarchy and the set of performance measures. Figure 4-2 illustrates how the value framework unites shared vision and shared leadership.

Feature 9: Culture of Community, Focused on Mission

Shared vision and shared leadership produce a culture of community, where all elements are fused into a coherent organization focused on the overall goal. *Culture of community* refers to social bonding of all members of the health care system. Transformation into a culture of community occurs in two ways:

1. The general management style is converted from authoritarian to participatory, with associated benefits of increased mutual respect, better morale, greater dedication among lower levels of management, and better ideas inserted into the management process.
2. Clearer focus on the central mission creates an esprit de corps where the focus has been on departmental issues and bureaucratization. The culture transforms from one that is at least partly bureaucratic into one with a mission that is shared institutionwide.

Other Useful Results of the Value Framework Process

The value framework process produces several other useful results. These include the values hierarchy, value communication devices, and a basis for communication.

The Values Hierarchy

A key output of the value framework process is the values hierarchy. A *values hierarchy* is a framework showing the many layers of the health care organization and how they interconnect to support the organization's vision. At the top is the organization's mission statement. Value performance measures become more specific with each lower layer. The lowest layer, or unit level, contains direct performance measures that provide guidance and incentives

Figure 4-2. Loading and Using the Value Framework

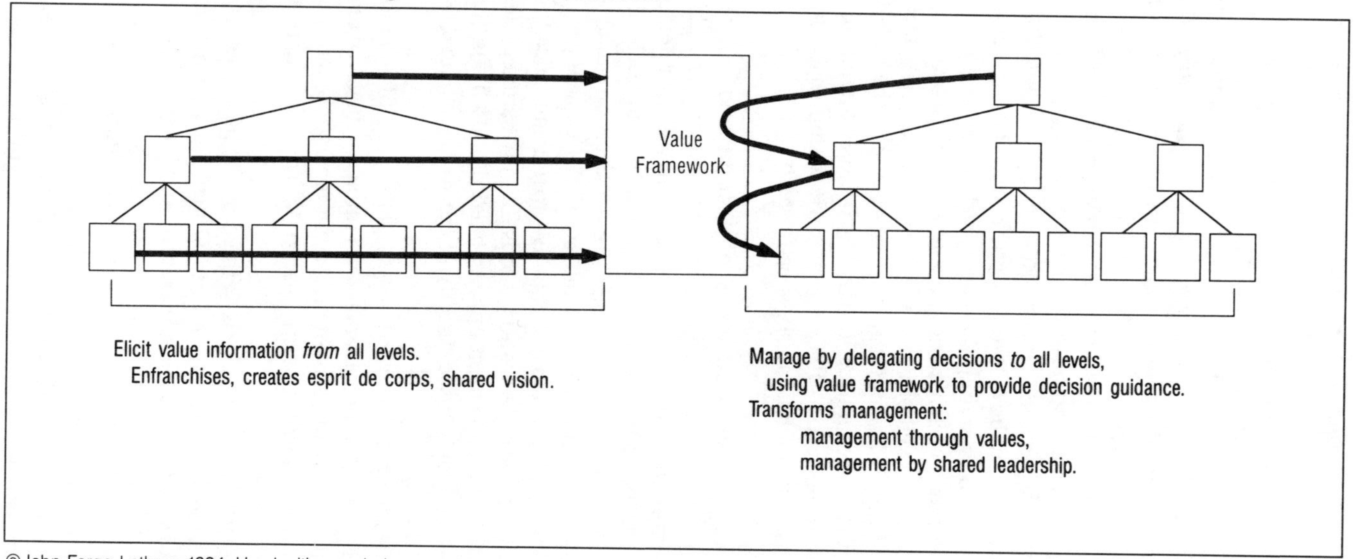
Value
Framework
Elicit value information *from* all levels.
Enfranchises, creates esprit de corps, shared vision.
Manage by delegating decisions *to* all levels,
using value framework to provide decision guidance.
Transforms management:
management through values,
management by shared leadership.

©John Fargo Lathrop 1994. Used with permission.

for operational decisions. These values are communicated in meaningful, practical terms.

Figure 4-3 presents an example values hierarchy. For brevity, only the high levels of that hierarchy are presented. For example, "work load" would be broken down into "professional" and "administrative," "professional" would then be broken down into "high affinity" and "low affinity," and so on. In a sense, there is only one "value" in figure 4-3 — the mission statement: effective community health care. All the rest of the hierarchy specifies the means to achieve that end. However, each of those means is individually important because we cannot directly predict how well each management decision will affect effective community health care. In fact, we do not even know how to directly measure the top value. Instead, we elicit value trade-offs among the lower-level values in order to assess their relative importance in achieving the highest-level value. It is important to note that without developing the values hierarchy, only a few of the values identified in figure 4-3 would come to mind. One of the benefits of a values hierarchy is that in generating it, typically broader overall values are identified and the more usual values are then fit within that context.

The values hierarchy has six specific features:

1. It provides a framework that ties together different levels of the institution, giving a shared vision for coherent action. The ability to define values within one consistent framework, from the strategic to the operational levels, not only uses inputs elicited from all levels of management but also provides outputs in the form of decision guidance and values definition/communication for all levels of management.
2. Higher layers of the values hierarchy provide guidance for decisions by defining what the organization stands for at the strategic level. The lower layers guide and implement operational decisions. Thus, the value framework process can be used directly in the strategic plan development and review process.
3. The values hierarchy provides many definitions of organizational value and thus provides a vocabulary — a common language for understanding — that can be useful in both internal communication and external communication of the institution's image to patients, providers, suppliers, and the service area.
4. Every layer of the hierarchy is defined by the layers below it. Every layer defines a single, concrete, and useful merit or performance measure to be optimized for decisions at that layer, using inputs from the layers below it.
5. The importance of any layer in the hierarchy is defined by the shared vision from that layer to the top layer.
6. Although this discussion has focused on a single hierarchy, in reality there may be several interlocking component hierarchies, each covering

Figure 4-3. Sample Values Hierarchy, High Levels Only

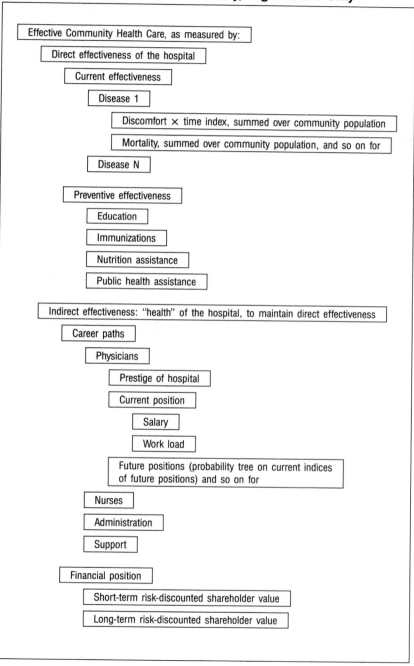

Effective Community Health Care, as measured by:

Direct effectiveness of the hospital

Current effectiveness

Disease 1

Discomfort × time index, summed over community population

Mortality, summed over community population, and so on for

Disease N

Preventive effectiveness

Education

Immunizations

Nutrition assistance

Public health assistance

Indirect effectiveness: "health" of the hospital, to maintain direct effectiveness

Career paths

Physicians

Prestige of hospital

Current position

Salary

Work load

Future positions (probability tree on current indices of future positions) and so on for

Nurses

Administration

Support

Financial position

Short-term risk-discounted shareholder value

Long-term risk-discounted shareholder value

a particular range of organizational levels and/or range of departments or other horizontal divisions, such as multihospital and care settings systems.

Value Communication Devices

Another useful result of the value framework process are value communication devices. *Value communication devices* are modifications of VDQs, which can be intermediate tools used to communicate values. Each VDQ can be converted into a value story, or parable, to illustrate particular value trade-offs between conflicting goals. Sets of these parables can be used to communicate value trade-offs of the organization to current, new, and prospective employees, patients, providers, suppliers, and the service area. Each class of recipient can receive a set of parables, selected to address the trade-offs most likely to be encountered by that recipient. For example, as an organization promotes a philosophy of patient-centeredness, departments within the organization will give up some of their individual decision making responsibilities. Disciplines from the many hospital departments will come together and learn to collaborate to achieve a common goal. They will move from a value of individual accountability to team accountability. This transition can be likened to geese flying in formation. Each goose plays a part in getting the whole flock to its destination. Geese take turns being leaders of the flock, supporting the entire flock in order that they reach the end of their journey. Publishing patient-related parables in the local paper would keep the institution and important health care value trade-offs in the public mind and demonstrate that the organization is thinking clearly and systematically about the value dilemmas with which it must deal, as well as preparing potential patients for trade-offs they may someday face in their own care.

Basis for Community Relations

The value framework process provides both a conceptual and concrete framework for a values-based public relations campaign with the community. *Conceptually,* the value structure cannot be developed by considering only the values within the institution; community input also is essential. The community must recognize that health care institutions cannot carry the complete burden of society's expectations for health care. Common ground must be reached between those expectations and the limitations of providing health care.

Concretely, the value structure can be communicated to the community during a strategically planned campaign that presents the institution's values and mission along with its limitations. This campaign could be called Managing Expectations. It would present the realities of health care in a way that dispels unrealistic notions as to what a health care system can provide under the current economic environment, and would feature clear and nondefensive explanations designed to enlist community understanding and cooperation. The public relations campaign could be presented at two levels. First, articles and announcements on the current health care situation and the institution's values and mission could be given to the press, repeating the same message in different forms: "Here is what we stand for. We are trying to meet your needs as much as humanly possible. Please work with us to achieve this. Here is how you can help." Second, actual examples of VDQs could be presented. For example: "Here is a patient situation. We can provide this specific care which probably will result in this outcome, in this amount of time, and at this expense but which carries with it these risks. Alternatively, we can provide different care, probably resulting in this outcome, quickly, at this expense, carrying additional risk. Both of these alternatives represent medical care performance that is well above national norms. Which would you choose?"

This type of campaign communicates important messages at three levels:

1. *We are a caring institution.* "We have a clear sense of the values involved in health care. Effective community health care is our paramount mission but there are limits as to what we can do. Family values are involved with decisions about appropriate care, and if you come to us, we will offer you choices so that our care can best meet your needs."
2. *Effective community health care is a matter of values: organizational values, community values, and the values of the patient and his or her family.* "As an organization/health care system, we are doing our share of bringing that care to you, but alone we cannot provide all the care you want at reasonable cost. You also have a role and responsibility in health care. We are all in this together."
3. *Health care is a matter of values and goals, not only of the health care system and the medical community but also of society as a whole.* "No amount of reworking of our hospital management or operations alone can meet the goals and aspirations society has for health care. As we adjust our own goals and operations to meet the new economic environment, we can achieve the goals society expects of us only if society makes adjustments in their goals and expectations as to what health care can accomplish. As an organization, we can help society make those adjustments by making our community aware of what can be achieved realistically, what the trade-offs are, and what the role and responsibilities of the individual are in his or her own health care. The clearer we are in these matters, the better we all will be able to achieve society's health care goals together."

• The Interactive Planning and Management Process

Most organizations undergoing successful transformation have come to recognize the advantage of using a defined management system to identify opportunities or goals for improvement and then to achieve them. Although many problem-solving or similar approaches may assist in this effort and result in success, the hospitals and systems in the SHNP found the principles of systems thinking in Senge's learning organization[2] and Ackoff's interactive planning model[3] to be most helpful. The *interactive planning and management process* is an interdisciplinary process built on systems thinking and design principles through which leaders and employees at all levels of the organization envision an organization's future and invent ways to achieve it.

Philosophical Foundation

Although commitment and active involvement by executives, directors, and managers are necessary to transform organizations, they cannot accomplish the change alone. Organizational transformation requires development of leaders followed by collaboration of leaders and followers (staff at all levels of the organization). Many who recognize the need for leadership fail not only to distinguish leadership from authority but also to recognize that leadership is the creation of "followership;" that is, leadership is a process requiring leaders and followers. Interactive planning and management focuses on leader–follower relationships, rather than on characteristics and traits of leadership. *Organizational transformation*, defined as fundamental change in how leaders and followers think, act, make decisions, and manage, calls for the design and practice of processes emphasizing the leader–follower relationship. When leaders and followers actively collaborate to develop shared vision and values, the experience is powerful and mobilizing. Collaborative efforts of leaders and followers demonstrate that the resulting vision and values are shared, and such initiatives move management into shared leadership. Managers are not transformed into leaders solely by executive decree. Exploring vision and values without the active leader–follower collaboration usually is a waste of time and resources, and can be destructive. Traditionally, vision and values are explored by a select group at the top of the organization and then handed down to lower levels for action. Such strategies need to be reframed from an approach based on authority and hierarchy to one of shared leadership based on leader–follower collaboration.

Leader–follower collaboration requires more time and effort, and appears messier and less efficient than change strategies based on authority and hierarchy. Consequently, many organizations choose authority-based strategies that constrain participation to avoid difference and conflict, even though the cost of these strategies is high and not readily apparent. With authority-based strategies, many fundamental issues are bypassed and energy for change remains external to the organization or is limited to only a part of it. This leads to organizational energy crisis and change agent burnout. The inefficiency of an authority-based strategy is eventually exposed by poor results and lack of desired outcomes.

Interactive planning and management is a change strategy and process in which leaders and followers collaborate and address differences and conflicts throughout the organization. It develops and renews organizational resources and personnel energy rather than depletes them. The process is used by some organizations to link vision and values with effective action planning, implementation and evaluation, and shared leadership; a different way of thinking and acting is built into day-to-day operational policy and practice.

Overview

Interactive planning differs significantly from two other commonly used types of planning: reactive and preactive. *Reactive planning* is tactically oriented and identifies deficiencies in the organization and then devises projects that remove them. *Preactive planning* is strategically oriented and consists of two major activities: predicting the future and preparing for it. This is based on the assumption that although the future is essentially uncontrollable, an organization with a good forecast of future environment is more likely to be able to control its effect. Preactive planning is concerned with planning *for* the future, not planning the future itself.

Interactive planning and management is directed at gaining control of the future. It is based on the belief that an organization's future depends at least as much on what it does between now and then as what is done to it. The design of a desirable future and the selection or intervention of ways to achieve it is termed *idealized design*. Idealized design has two stages: idealization and realization. Idealization consists of planning and design, and realization consists of invention and management. The name *interactive planning and management* connotes that these stages have a systemic interrelationship that should never be separated in organizational practice, which is often common practice. The two stages have five interrelated phases (as shown in figure 4-4):

1. The idealization stage
   - *Phase 1: situational analysis.* Every organization is faced with interrelated problems and opportunities. This phase determines the pattern of interaction among these problems and opportunities and identifies the constraints that prevent solution. The result is a formulation of the current system of problems, or "the mess."

Figure 4-4.   The Interactive Planning and Management Process

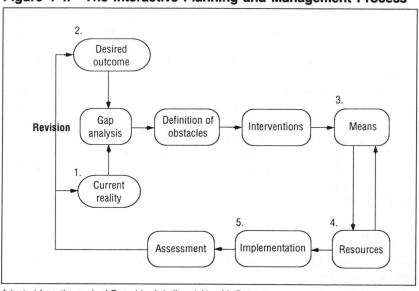

Adapted from the work of Russel L. Ackoff and Alan M. Barstow

- *Phase 2: ends planning.* This phase articulates the organization's desired future by means of the idealized design process. Goals, objectives, and ideals are defined. By comparing the current situation and the idealized design, the gaps to be closed or narrowed by the planning process are identified.
2. The realization stage
   - *Phase 3: means planning.* What should be done to close or narrow the gaps identified in ends planning is defined, including assessment of the obstacles and the selection of intervention for appropriate courses of action, practices, projects, programs, and policies.
   - *Phase 4: resources planning.* The type and amount of resources required, when they will be required, and how are they to be acquired or generated are determined.
   - *Phase 5: implementation and control.* The organization specifies who is to do what and when each task is to be performed, as well as a means of assessing results, that is, assignments and schedules are carried out as expected and produce the desired effects on performance.

Revision and celebration will start the process over as not only will current reality be altered, but also a new desired outcome may be evident. The five phases of interactive planning and management usually are initiated in this order, although they need not be. Because they are strongly interdependent, they generally are implemented simultaneously and interactively. In continuous planning, no phase is finally completed; all outputs are subject to subsequent revision.

During these phases, designers of the process assume that the organization has been completely destroyed, even though its environment has remained unchanged. The ensuing design effort is directed at replacing the existing organization with one that would operate in the current environment as opposed to a forecasted one. Constraints placed on the idealized design are that it be:

- *Technologically feasible:* The design cannot rely on unproven technology, although available technologies can be used in new ways. This constraint prevents the design process from becoming an exercise in science fiction.
- *Operationally viable:* The new organization should be capable of surviving in the current environment if it were brought into existence today. Designers must focus on viability in today's environment. Full participation in the idealized design process enlarges the conception of what can be implemented, and acknowledgment or discussion of obstacles perceived at this stage will be detrimental.
- *Capable of rapid learning and adaptation:* An organization is a voluntary association of purposeful members, and it cannot operate effectively independent of their desires and values. Additionally, every organization is part of a larger environment that also is purposeful. Therefore, the organization should be capable of adjusting itself as the values of its members and the requirements of its environment change. This translates into the following subrequirements:
  - The stakeholders of the organization should be able to modify the design at any time because their knowledge, understanding, and values change, especially as a result of efforts to realize the design.
  - Design conflicts that cannot be settled by consensus are handled by incorporating processes for reexamination and rediscussion into the experimental design of the organization. This enables the organization to learn continuously from its own experience and to improve itself over time.
  - Decisions and the critical assumptions on which they are based should be subject to control. The expected effects of each decision, the time by which they are expected, and the assumptions on which these decisions are based should be formulated and monitored. When they deviate significantly from the actual effects or conditions, corrective action is taken where appropriate.

The product of an idealized design is not an ideal system. Rather, it is a system that can be improved by its designers and is capable of improving itself. It is the best ideal-seeking system that its designers can conceive now.

Characteristics of the idealized design process emphasize its interactive nature. Those characteristics are:

- *Participation:* Most system redesign is assigned to experts because effort is directed at identifying and correcting deficiencies of an existing system. This requires specific knowledge of the system's structure and function. In idealized design, the existing system is irrelevant and focus is on what the system ought to be, rather than on what can be made of it as it now exists. Those directly affected by a system — its stakeholders — are the experts who can determine what the system ought to be. Each is qualified to express opinion on how the organization should operate. Individual stakeholders tend to focus on different aspects of the system and as many of them as possible should be involved to ensure that all aspects are considered. The redesign of these aspects will be synthesized into one design characterized by a depth and comprehensiveness that no external consultant can provide, because stakeholders who have been immersed in the operation of components have a better understanding of how they interact than do any outside experts. Stakeholders learn about the system during the idealized design process, particularly about how interaction of the parts affects overall performance. This enables them to shift focus and concern from one part, which is "theirs," to recognize and be concerned with how it affects other parts, and ultimately, the whole.
- *Consensus:* The idealized design process generates consensus among participants who disagree less on ideals than on the means to be used to pursue them. Because of this, individual differences over means are more easily resolved. When differences cannot be resolved, participants need only agree on the design of criteria to resolve them and agreement is easier to obtain.
- *Commitment:* Participation and consensus produce commitment. Participants are more strongly committed to ideas they developed themselves than they are to ideas handed down to them. Participation reduces problems associated not only with selling an idea to others but also in achieving commitment to cooperate in its implementation.
- *Creativity:* One process of inducing creativity consists of identifying self-imposed constraints, relaxing or removing them, and exploring new possibilities without them. Because the idealized design process assumes that the current system no longer exists, many of the self-imposed constraints that operate when existing system improvement is attempted by removing deficiencies are removed. Additionally, because destruction of the organization is imaginary, the design process for the participants is fun and imaginative creativity is liberated.
- *Feasibility:* A principal obstruction to creativity is preoccupation with feasibility. This constraint is removed in idealized design because the participants' conception of feasibility usually undergoes major revision in

the process. In conventional system design, estimates of feasibility are inferred from estimates of feasibility of parts taken separately. Like a chain, such design is limited and is only as feasible as its least feasible link. However, an idealized design is a system of decisions. It is possible to produce a feasible idealized design, none of whose parts taken separately is feasible. Conversely, it is possible to have an infeasible idealized design each of whose parts, if taken separately, is feasible.

The Steps of the Process

Although the organization must make an informed decision as to whether to engage in interactive planning and management, this is not the first step. The first step is education. Because the system as a whole should be involved in making the decision to become involved in interactive planning and management, and not just the CEO or the executive committee, the entire organization should be introduced to the process and educated about its principles and practices. Many health care organizations were exposed to the principles of interactive planning and systems thinking through nationally presented programs sponsored by professional organizations. SHNP also provided a general learning session for the project teams participating in the national initiative. Executives interested in this strategy and process then sponsored educational sessions that were attended by people from all levels and departments of the organization mixed together. The sessions were interactive, not lectures. The ideal is to get the whole system in one room, exposing as many people as possible to interactive planning and management, and give them the opportunity to compare and contrast this process to other approaches, including organizational customs and habits. Participants in these facilitated sessions discuss the process, express their doubts and hopes, and listen to the concerns and desires of others, thereby developing a deeper, shared understanding of the process. This is the foundation on which the organization can make an informed decision about participation, and can enlist commitment to the process. The next steps are to provide integration and coordination throughout the organization by establishing:

- *An interactive planning task force to launch the process:* This is a temporary work group formed to undertake support of the change effort. It should include seven to nine members, chosen from different levels of the organization. Thoughtful selection of members is critical and should include senior-level leadership and frontline managers, along with physicians and other caregivers. The task force engages the stakeholders in dialogue in order to discover common ground and commit the organization to action. It does most of the work of developing the situational analysis and the idealized design, which leads to identification of interventions that are used to realize desired outcomes.

- *An interactive planning council to communicate effectively with the entire organization and its stakeholders:* The council is a large group of stakeholders who need to be kept informed and involved in the change effort and to whom the task force presents its findings and recommendations. Ideally, representatives from the whole system, including all levels of management and care providers with members of the board of trustees, are selected to meet together in one room to engage in dialogue. Although this is impossible logistically, it is desirable in principle. As with the task force, this critical process results in discovery of common ground and shared commitment to act. All members of the organization are kept informed of council outcomes. The council can serve as the primary decision-making body for the organization, referring recommendations and actions to executive leaders and the board of trustees.
- *A system of planning and management boards to build the process into the organization and sustain it as standard operating procedure:* An interlinking system of planning and management boards is established to close the gap between the current situation and the idealized design, as well as to provide a basis for practice of the interactive planning and management process throughout the organization (that is, their responsibility is to transform the planning and idealization that comes from the task force and council into management policy and realization). Membership on these boards provides an effective means of shared leadership and collaboration not only in managing the present situation but also in creating the future. The boards increase the readiness, willingness, and ability of the organization to change. They are based on the principle that those who are directly affected by a decision should be involved in the decision-making process and that the quality of decisions is improved when multiple perspectives are focused on an issue. Every manager in the organization has a board and every board consists of the manager, the manager's boss, and the manager's direct reports. Three management levels on each board ensures effective vertical integration. In most cases, boards also include other stakeholders to enhance horizontal coordination within the organization. As a result, boards throughout the organization overlap and interlink, making them extremely effective in sharing information and managing interactions between units and departments. Initially, the boards meet frequently, perhaps once a week, to get started and build momentum. As the process continues, they meet monthly, with occasional periods of intensified activity. The interlinking system of boards thus becomes the vehicle for iterative cycles of interactive planning and management for the continuous redesign and improvement of the organization. This interlinking design is often referred to as *circular* and is supportive of collaborative management models for institutional decision making.[4] This structure can replace traditional hierarchical decision making and transition the organization to an interactive, participative structure for realizing both operational and clinical opportunities.

Interactive planning and management is a lever for realizing effective change. It enables the organization to redesign, renew, and revitalize itself rather than reactively fix problems and treat symptoms. Through this continuous change process, organization members—both leaders and followers—collaborate to envision a desirable future and close the gap between this future and their current situation.

• Conclusion

Transformational leaders encourage and inspire their organizations to develop a shared vision and to move toward shared leadership. Using processes such as the value framework and interactive planning and management, leaders define values and manage through participation with stakeholders throughout the entire organization. All decisions, from strategic planning to the multitude of decentralized decisions made at all levels of the institution, can be made by applying guidance from either or both of these processes. The net effect is that every level of decision maker, down to unit staff, understands the institution's values, opportunities, and desired outcomes well enough to make his or her own decisions, but make them in alignment with the rest of the organization. In that way, those closest to the work are empowered to make decisions that allow them to work in the most efficient and cost-effective way.

The value framework process is based on a values hierarchy, where each layer of the hierarchy is a set of performance measures that define a value or goal in subjective but quantitative terms. The process of setting up the value framework consults all levels of organizational management and builds mutual empathy, trust, and respect among all members of the organization. It creates an esprit de corps and shared vision across all levels. The interactive planning and management process is based on criteria that define the best ideal-seeking system that its designers can conceive. It is constrained only by what is technically feasible, operationally viable, and capable of rapid learning and adaption. The framework and the interactive process provide explicit guidance for decision making at all levels. Both processes require leaders and followers to actively collaborate in developing a shared vision and values, and both move stakeholders toward shared leadership. They are useful methods for communicating values, both internally and externally; for maintaining consistency among delegated decisions; for identifying resolutions to conflicts and solutions to problems; and for enabling better coordination among departments. The desired outcome of both processes is to transform the organization into a culture of community.

References and Note

1. Delbecq, A. L., Van de Ven, A. H., and Gustafson, D. H. *Techniques and Program Planning: A Guide to Nominal Group Technique and Delphi Process.* Glenview, IL: Scott Foresman, 1975.

2. Senge, P. M. *The Fifth Discipline: The Art and Practice of the Learning Organization.* New York City: Doubleday, 1990.

3. Ackoff, R. L. *Creating the Corporate Future.* New York City: John Wiley and Sons, 1981.

4. For more information on the concept of the circular organization and planning and management boards, see: Ackoff, R. L. *Creating the Corporate Future.* New York City: John Wiley and Sons, 1981; and the Academy of Management. *Executive* 3(1):11–16, 1989.

Chapter 5

Making the Change

The Teacher is like the Shadow; always there, but never an encumbrance. Who can catch the Shadow? What we learn becomes the Shadow. We are first the student, then we become our own teacher.

Lightningbolt, Hyemeyohsts Storm

The sound and fury of an individual's creative life are the elemental waters missing from the dehydrated workday. The frightening emptiness of existence also contains a place of nourishment and repose, a blessed opportunity for calm at the center of the corporate whirlwind. . . . Adaptability and native creativity on the part of the workforce come through the door only with their passions. Their passions come only with their souls. Their souls love the hidden springs boiling and welling at the center of existence more than they love the company.

The Heart Aroused: Poetry and the Preservation of the Soul in Corporate America, David Whyte

Change is difficult for both individuals and organizations. When an organization is undergoing change, its environment becomes unfamiliar and uncomfortable. Often people respond to the uncertainty that change brings by objecting to change, complaining about it, blaming others for it, or denying that it is needed. Some respond to change by leaving the organization. Accepting change often requires reexamination of self—both individual and organizational self—and stretching prior limits and boundaries, which can be a painful process. As new skills and capabilities evolve, different patterns of thinking, seeing, and behaving emerge. For example, the tendency to immediately blame an inefficiency on someone or something becomes tempered by new patience, awareness, insight, and sensibility on the part of the forces that affect that situation. Organizations that have been successful in the change process have leaders who not only live the vision, but also teach, mentor, and coach the process of implementing that vision, encouraging others to stretch and grow. Such leaders are able to actualize the destiny of their organization within the community.

This chapter examines the phenomenon of the "Ah ha" experience through the voices of transformational leaders who have made the transition to change.

• "Ah Ha" Experiences

"Ah ha" experiences are those moments when individuals in the throes of organizational transformation gain personal insights that change their beliefs and behaviors. Such experiences may come suddenly or gradually as new knowledge is assimilated. As pupils become teachers to others, and institutional implementation of organizational interaction through processes such as the value framework process and/or the interactive planning and management process proceed, a definite and palpable change occurs. Those who have undergone such experiences often describe them in spiritual terms. For example, this point in organizational transformation sometimes is called "the birth of the organizational soul." When individuals realize their personal goals are aligned with institutional goals, a sense of shared destiny is experienced, and new energy and motivation permeate the organization.

During the transition to change, the organization's most important resource — its people — must be empowered, meaning they must be taught to become self-directed and allowed to participate in the decisions that affect their working life. With the accelerated rate of change in health care today, self-direction becomes an imperative.[1,2] Tearing down the hierarchy that limits communications, adaptability, and responsiveness is essential. This means providing people with means for self-direction, allowing them to experience possibilities for collaboration, to cultivate their imagination, and to use their intuition to create the means to improve the value of patient care for their community.

In *Lightningbolt,* Storm says that "the greatest battle in life is subtle. The reality of Self ignorance is obvious to the learned, but the person who is ignorant cannot see the truth about the Self. The ignorant seek to conform."[3] Traditionally, health care has been built on seeking to conform and compete, rather than on discovering the reason for our existence by working together, learning from each other, and becoming cocreators in building a better health care system for our community. The ability to build on tradition while shifting to new insights, awarenesses, and sensibilities is what distinguishes transformational leaders. Transformational leaders respect themselves and at the same time recognize the importance of instilling self-direction in others. They understand that they are first the student and then the teacher whose mission is to invest in the talent, imagination, and creativity of everyone at every level in the organization. Their desired outcomes are both personal and professional, interconnecting dimensions for the good of the patient, the organization, and the community.

Thus, organizational change starts with a dream that evolves into a shared vision and belief by everyone linked with the organization's destiny. It is built on sound strategy with planning and implementation processes and integrated infrastructures appropriate to those strategies. And most important, it is built on the talents, knowledge, and skills of the people within the organization and the community.[4]

• Transformational Leaders on "Ah Ha" Experiences

Sharing personal experiences that bring new insights and shift beliefs and behaviors is meaningful for both self-learning and team learning. Following are examples of insightful moments, new awarenesses, and the shift to new sensibilities as described by transformational leaders in a variety of institutions. Their experiences are grouped as follows:

- Getting beyond traditional assumptions and practices
- Redesigning roles and structure
- Overcoming barriers to change

Getting beyond Traditional Assumptions and Practices

The following transformational leaders gained insights that enabled them to more fully recognize the contributions and perspectives of others at different levels of the organization, both staff and patients, and to accept their participation as members of the care delivery team.

Richard Lindsay, head, division of geriatric medicine, University of Virginia: The title of the Strengthening Hospital Nursing Program (SHNP) surfaced some of the long-standing differences between medicine and nursing. Along with other advisory committee members, I felt this program would create dissention about strengthening nursing rather than improving the outcome of patient care. I asked myself: "Do nurses really need to be given more power? Isn't the issue more that nurses are too far away from direct patient care?" My previous experience with nursing was from my specialty of geriatric medicine. Team participation and input from everyone, including the patient and the family, is standard practice for managing the geriatric patient and the family of the patient, and I felt that more administrative responsibility for the nurse would only detract from that primary role. I now understand the narrowness of my knowledge at that time about the proper role nursing plays in providing effective and appropriate patient care services. Nurses are essential members not only of the decision-making team deciding about the plan of care, but also in deciding about the efficiencies and efficaciousness of the care itself. They play that same important role with all patient care services, and it is precisely that participatory practice that is central to the restructuring objectives of the SHNP, rather than furnishing nursing more power or administrative responsibility. The nonphysician, nonnursing members of the advisory committee demonstrated to the professional members that the traditional way of caring for patients was ineffective, and the goal of SHNP was not just about governance, but it more importantly was about patient care with effective utilization of professional resources through teamwork. It was this participation in the advisory committee discussions that led to my own personal "insight" and encouraged me to greatly expand my awareness of the role of nursing. This same issue surfaced with many of the participating institutions, and one of the major ingredients in the success of SHNP was the creation of an awareness that the project was about improving patient care, rather than giving nurses more power.

Brad Brown, vice-president, management information systems, Tallahassee Memorial Regional Medical Center: "Why are we doing this thing called redesign? We know how to do our jobs!" This theme echoed through the hallways of our management information services department as our hospital entered Startup, a six-month process to train hospital workers to redesign work using the interactive management and planning process. Not realizing what this change ultimately would mean to the organization, we did not focus initially on the why of change, but on the how of change. As a result, each person achieved a realization of the impact of this process in different ways. Some remained trapped in old paradigms, while others made the connection, but only after some gut-wrenching experiences. The following scenario demonstrates the significance of starting with the why of change. It also shows a moment of new awareness, an "Ah ha" for the young woman involved — and for me.

Well into the development of the idealized design, Ms. A came to me and asked to be taken out of Startup. She said, "I don't understand where we're going and I don't understand how it's going to help me. I frankly think it's a waste of my time." Trying to explain how it would help her feel more empowered and more involved in the mission of the hospital, I received a blank stare in return. At that moment, I realized my buzzwords and terminology were words with no apparent link to her reality. She could not identify with these concepts because she had no point of reference. We went to the chalkboard for a conversation about her concerns. She was asked to list things she liked about her job and things she disliked. After completing the lists, she was asked to check those items she could influence or change. She could not check even one item, stating, "Those things are out of my control." She could not see herself changing the environment because she felt powerless, and she did not understand why she needed to change the way she did her work. During our discussion, we created the philosophy of *you*:

- *You,* if you are affected, have the right to know and understand why change is needed.
- *You* have the power and responsibility to make changes which affect your work.
- *You* have the power and responsibility to influence the direction of the organization.
- *You* have the power and responsibility to involve others (stakeholders) in support of that direction.

Planning how this philosophy could be implemented via the planning boards, a new awareness dawned for both of us. For Ms. A, it was the realization that the process itself was empowerment, not just an abstract concept. By "doing it," she understood and "embraced it." For me, it was an equally dramatic insight as I realized I would need to be willing to relinquish authority to the staff and learn to facilitate and coach, instead of dictate and supervise. Above all, I would need to instill the same willingness in my entire management staff. I have learned that leaders who listen to the ideas of their employees and provide an interactive feedback mechanism holding them accountable for results will achieve rewards beyond what they could do within traditional top-down decision-making systems.

Sharon Lee, vice-president, patient care services, St. Luke's Regional Medical Center: It is important to realize that no one person has 100 percent responsibility or control of what needs to happen to create a better environment. We each should acknowledge and take responsibility for what we can contribute. We must be open, proactive, and creative, allowing flexibility where indicated and accepting the part of others in the work that must be accomplished for change to occur. Understanding one's own values, experiences, and attitudes will bring about a change in how we deal with change. When I understood and accepted this about myself, I could make the personal shift to change my leadership style and help others to do the same.

William Manahan, medical director of quality assurance, Immanuel-St. Joseph's Hospital: I was brought up in a system where I was taught that those at the top generally, if not always, knew what was best for me. This group includes parents, teachers, church officials, coaches, bosses, and law enforcement officials. There is truth to this concept for all of us at a young age, and even for some of us at other times in our life. However, if we want to learn about ourselves at the deepest level, we often need to follow our own instinct and beliefs, and not those of someone else. We need to change our way of thinking from a top-down model to trusting ourselves and ultimately trusting others. From that point, it is only a short jump to realize that to make our own decisions, we should have as much input as possible. Teamwork and collaborative thinking help to make better decisions for everyone involved.

Probably the closest "Ah ha" experience for me can be illustrated in the following experience. Having an interest in preventive medicine and patient responsibility, I often spent quite a bit of time in educating my patients in ways that would be helpful to prevent the problem for which they were seeing me. I thought that I, as the doctor, knew what was right for the patient. Gradually, I learned that a large number of patients did not take my advice and those that did often were unable to maintain the changed behavior. The patient now had an added burden of guilt about not being able to follow through on what they had started (quitting smoking, exercising, or changing their diet). I learned that much more than knowledge was needed to make significant change. There had to be an attitude of wanting to make the change, and there had to be the learning of skills on how to make the change. It was at that moment that I realized that I had only been giving my patients one third of what they needed to make their changes. Knowledge was not enough. I also needed to help them with skills and attitude changes. I began to ask my patients what they thought about making the change. If they were not eager to do it, I would then explore with them other avenues and ideas that might help them with the problem. The exciting thing about accepting the perspective of the patient means that instead of walking out of the exam room with what felt like a lose-lose situation (I felt bad because I had scolded the patient, and the patient felt shamed because they were scolded), we walked out feeling it was a win-win for both of us. The patient had something that he or she had suggested working on, and I felt good about guiding the patient to do what he or she thought needed to be done, instead of scolding them.

This type of experience is what transformational leadership is really about. Even when the leaders of a hospital are sure they know what needs to be done or know what is best for the organization, it does not necessarily mean that it can be imposed from above with any kind of success. In most instances, better success will be obtained by collaborating with the involved players in a search for a workable solution. Transforming the style of leadership means that leaders will develop a system in which those who are closest to the work will be provided guidance on the best ways to do the work that needs to be done. In other words, I see it as more of a horizontal than a vertical or top-down system, a system where people (employees and other concerned parties) are empowered (which only they can do themselves) to feel a share in and a responsibility for the larger organization and for the broader community.

Redesigning Roles and Structure

The following transformational leaders describe their response to the redefinition of roles, including their own, brought about by organizational transformation.

Linda Fleury, human resource analyst, MeritCare Health System: To support management and staff in coping with the fast and constant changes occurring in the health care environment, human resources (HR) has to be flexible and adaptable. We have changed our organizational structure, placing the customer (patient) at the top, rather than at the bottom of the usual hierarchy of administration. The traditional role of HR being administrative record keepers no longer meets the needs of an organization that is patient needs responsive. Management is challenged with reengineering how work is being done, determining who has the skills to meet the needs of the customer, and rewarding managers and staff who produce results. HR must become more self-directed and assume the role of internal consultant, providing knowledge and skills to help managers through these challenges. If we accept the challenge of developing the work force, I believe that we can do more with less, and maintain high-quality, patient-centered services that are cost-effective.

Annette Compton, director of volunteers, St. Luke's Regional Medical Center: As the leader of St. Luke's Regional Medical Center's work group on redesigning the system for the delivery of nonclinical services, I could see that the only way we could achieve our goal was to completely redesign all of our systems and remove the barriers to progress. This was my first indication that roles, including my own, needed to change. The second was the rapidly changing reports on the finances of the hospital. Low patient census, shorter patient stays, and increase of outpatient procedures clearly indicated a need to reduce our cost. These changes seemed to occur so fast and were difficult to understand, but it was evident we needed to redesign our system so fewer employees were doing the work more efficiently.

Sharon Lee, vice-president, patient care services, St. Luke's Regional Medical Center: Hospitals must meet the challenge of restructuring care delivery and management systems in order to meet the quality/cost balance in a transformed payment environment. Over the past few years, it has become apparent to our leadership that we cannot achieve that balance without redesigning roles and structure throughout the organization. To do less only asks individuals to do the same work with fewer staff. Over time, that would have an adverse impact on the quality of care that we deliver. As St. Luke's Medical Center's design team began to work on the concept of patient-centered care, with the intent of eliminating traditional department structures and placing clinicians in interdisciplinary teams at the unit level, it was obvious that the entire organization, including organizational and departmental management, would have to undergo the same radical transformation. Leadership cannot ask others to change their roles, putting their professional values and traditions at risk, without being willing to do the same. Management structure and roles need to change before others could be asked to change. In fact, we believe this is an essential step in order to have the appropriate support structure for change to take place. Otherwise, there are incentives to keep things the way they are, in order to protect self.

It is important for everyone to realize their choices during times of change. This can prevent them from feeling like a victim to the change.

Understanding our ability to have choices, we can talk in terms of what we could do rather than what we couldn't or wouldn't do. That, in itself, becomes freeing — a step toward healing and toward the change that needs to happen.

William Manahan, medical director of quality assurance, Immanuel-St. Joseph's Hospital: A hierarchical system does not honor and respect the worth and dignity of every person. The underlying message of that system is that I, the leader, know what is best for you. This does not mean that the leader never gives directions or says what needs to be done, but that when possible, input from all involved people is obtained and incorporated into the plan for action. Doing this elicits the innate intelligence and self-worth of every person involved. It is a commitment and a deep faith that we are all an extension of each other, and the greater good will be served for all of us.

How this applies to my role . . . is demonstrated in the following example: Physicians were complaining that they were not receiving information soon enough on patients who had been in the emergency department the previous few days. Those patients would go to their doctor's office for follow-up, and there would be no record of what had happened in the ER. Using a vertical style of leadership (as I probably would have done in the past), I would have gone to the emergency room physicians and told them they had to have all patient charts dictated before they left the hospital at the end of their shift. I then would have gone to medical records and told the director that the maximum turnover time for emergency room dictations was to be 24 hours or less. Even though these changes might have solved the problem if implemented, a tremendous amount of resistance both from the emergency room physicians and from the medical record personnel could be expected, based on past experience. Based on the transformational style of leadership, a team was formed to study the problem and made recommendations. The director of medical records stated that she was unable to hire good medical record transcriptionists because of a shortage in most rural areas of competent medical transcriptionists. Hospital administration said they would be willing to budget immediately to send the dictations to a consulting service, and that would give us a 24-hour turnaround time. The medical record department started training their own transcriptionists to ensure an adequate supply locally in the future. These measures solved the delay in transcription time dramatically and easily. When the emergency room physician dictation times were evaluated, it was evident that only two of the five emergency room physicians did not dictate their charts by the end of their shift. Because of their style of seeing patients, they felt they were unable to do all the dictations by the end of their shift. A compromise was reached in that all pertinent information would be handwritten by them on the ER sheet at the time of the patient visit. That sheet would then go to the physician's office, and those two physicians would dictate later to ensure a more complete and more legal medical record. This system seemed to work well, and both the emergency room physicians and the local physicians were satisfied with the outcome. This example demonstrates that when key stakeholders become involved in a task force, appropriate data are obtained, recommendations are made, and since the recommendations are made by the people involved, they are followed appropriately. This style of transformational leadership just makes good sense.

Overcoming Barriers to Change

The following transformational leaders discuss their perspectives on the barriers within their institutions to implementing organizational transformation, including the barriers they themselves present.

Linda Fleury, human resource analyst, MeritCare Health System: There are two barriers to implementing organizational change: (1) lack of skills and training to be effective in a new leadership role, and (2) top-management support for the role of internal consultant. When new ideas are initiated, outside consultants usually are pursued instead of giving the opportunity to internal staff and instilling confidence in them to do an effective job.

Annette Compton, director of volunteers, St. Luke's Regional Medical Center: As is often the case, we are our own worse enemy. I am probably my greatest barrier. I've always greeted change as an opportunity, but giving up the old has been difficult. It was hard to see capable people leave, many of whom had become good friends. I worried of what would happen if our most capable people all left. The local press headlined our actions incorrectly and I spent much of my time explaining the hospital's actions. The media made it difficult for those of us who interfaced with the community and difficult for employees who were getting mixed messages. I hadn't anticipated this, and initially I found myself being reactive instead of proactive.

Sharon Lee, vice-president, patient care services, St. Luke's Regional Medical Center: After overcoming the barrier that was within myself, I was able to focus on opportunities and on the job at hand, and begin to develop new relationships with a different, expanded group of staff. New trust relationships need to be developed. Obviously this will take place over time as systems are changed and as individuals find their place in the new system and structure. We have eliminated functional departments as they existed and have implemented services to erase departmental barriers. However, professional and technical territoriality continue to exist. I believe that these, too, will be overcome with time, as my role and the roles of others are cemented.

Barriers that affect my role as facilitator of the change process include the changing environment and health care financing. Change is difficult enough in a stable environment. However, it is even more difficult in an environment that is changing at a rapid pace with an uncertain outcome. With the financial future as uncertain as it is, along with the decrease in patient days and length of stay, the budget is a moving target. There is increased pressure for high levels of productivity and to accomplish the same level of work with fewer staff. We are faced with the imperative of reducing our work force by the end of our current fiscal year. We all know that the work has to be restructured in order to gain the economies desired, but that takes a commitment of resources to effect the change. The barrier becomes the trade-off of time spent delivering patient care or time spent planning for the changes and their implementation. In addition, we are dealing with employee fear that we will be having a layoff, a paralyzing thought in these critical times. While we are striving to accomplish our reductions through a combination of attrition, voluntary separation, and early retirement incentive plans, the fear continues and will most likely not abate until the restructure is complete and all of the outcomes are known. This is a catch-22. We know, and the employees know, that the restructure will result in the need for fewer staff, a factor that does not provide incentive for staff assistance in the changes required to stay strong for the future challenges that we face. This requires a significant amount of communication, strategizing, and consensus building to prioritize what needs to be done and when it needs to be done in order to achieve our vision and goals. It requires teamwork from a team that hasn't reached the point of performing as a team, since everyone has had a role change and no one is totally comfortable in their new role as yet.

William Manahan, medical director of quality assurance, Immanuel-St. Joseph's Hospital: Barriers include my need to be in charge, my need to control, and the belief that I truly know what is best for other people. There is a lack of confidence that if I let go and really trust other people, it won't be done well enough.

Edward Foley, regional vice-president, Hospital of Southern California: Barriers include my concern with my own self-image to the physician community, to my corporate colleagues, and (since I was in a publicly owned hospital) the entire political arena. People in the community expect, and in some cases demand, predictability from their colleagues and leaders. Change is apt to be very unsettling. Thus, a great deal of time and attention must be paid to helping these audiences see the merit, the appropriateness, and the requirement for your own change. They know this change in your program and behavior will have an affect on them. They need to be reassured good outcomes will flow from these changes, even though there may be some rocky moments during the transition. Success with these groups is critically important; any one of them could torpedo your plans and even zap your career.

• Case Study: Hackley Hospital

An example of a health care organization that has successfully initiated its transformation is Hackley Hospital, in Muskegon, Michigan. The hospital received two awards in 1994: The Muskegon, MI, County Quality Award and the 21st Century Innovators Award, sponsored by The Health Care Forum and 3M. Thomas Mroczkowski, vide president/COO, explains how Hackley Hospital did it:

Two occurrences come to mind as I think about building a vision and commitment to change. The first was in 1987 and the other was in 1992. In 1987, having been promoted from a division head to chief operating officer, it became apparent, while the clinical side of health care was advancing at an increasingly rapid rate, the leadership side was stagnant, showing no significant change or improvement in many years. This situation was even more obvious when I compared health care to other industries. It was my belief that the bureaucratic style of health care leadership needed to transform into a more participative and team-oriented approach. My role had to change from boss to team leader. There were many challenges to make this change a reality, including meeting the expectations of the management group. I found that there was a tremendous organizational culture difference between the authoritarian, bureaucratic style and the participative, team style of leadership. Critical elements such as shared vision, focused objectives, teamwork, and shared decision making often receive lip service in a bureaucratic environment, but are essential in the new team-based system. Old habits, patterns of behavior, and mental models were significant barriers that interfered with this change. Turf issues and departmental conflict further complicated the transformation.

Positive factors included a board and CEO who understood and supported the need for change and a medical staff that was generally contemporary and willing to listen to new ideas. Because of the magnitude of this change, possibly one of the most significant ever undertaken by the organization, it became apparent that this could not be completely internally driven. We looked for an external change agent, and selected a management consultant to serve in this role. Shortly after initiating the change process, we received the SHNP planning award. The education, training, and guidance received through this program supported and enhanced our efforts. For example, the exposure to the work of Russell Ackoff. His idealized redesign and planning board concepts were implemented as the foundation of our new participative leadership style. These events, along with much additional research and educational opportunities, gave credibility to the transformation process experienced by the hospital. It provided credibility to my new participative leadership role, which has served as an acceptable leadership model for others to emulate.

The path that we chose has proven to be right and appropriate. The organization will continue to evolve along the lines of empowerment, cross-functional work teams, and shared decision making. For myself,

I need to become more adept at consensus building and facilitation among diverse constituencies. These are probably some of the most essential skills needed to achieve results within this new leadership paradigm. For the organization, we need to continue to refine processes and systems that enable further erosion of the walls and barriers that still stand in the way of achieving our objectives in the most effective and efficient manner possible. For example, we are promoting a future organization that includes only four general groupings:

- Clinical information, such as the lab, radiology, physiology
- Direct caregivers, such as nursing, physical therapy, and occupational therapy
- Hospitality services, such as food, housekeeping, maintenance
- Administrative support or business services

In our new model, other departmental distinctions do not serve a meaningful purpose as separate entities. In fact, maintaining their separateness is viewed as a barrier towards achieving our patient care objectives in the most optimal manner possible.

There are significant times when one has a unique insight or new awareness. This is probably a necessary precursor to change of any significance. At some point, diverse and seemingly unrelated events come together at a point in time when everything just seems to make sense. For me, it was a feeling of absolute certainty that this new course of action was absolutely the right one. The most recent visioning process occurred in 1992. It was fascinating to me to note that, while it definitely built on my earlier beliefs, this vision has a different emphasis, although I experienced similar developmental stages. This "Ah ha" experience concerns health care reform, redefining the very function and purpose of hospitals and health care institutions. It involves understanding that medical care is not health care, meaning that health care includes many dimensions of health status such as housing, crime, nutrition, lifestyle, and preventive care. This belief is changing our emphasis from an inward-directed medical care facility, to an outward-focused community participant, offering special skills and services directed toward improving the health status of our community. To become more involved with this movement, I served in a year-long Creating Healthier Communities fellowship offered by the Healthcare Forum. My project for the fellowship is based on the premise that the total health care needs of a majority of the population in our communities are not being met to varying degrees. This includes availability, both medical and health care, regardless of the socioeconomic status of the individual. It is the goal of Hackley Hospital to participate in operationalizing many of the principles from Creating Healthier Communities fellowship. Market forces are driving physician–hospital affiliations and, while this integration is positive, such partnerships alone will not significantly impact health status. Paramount to redefining health is education as well as building support structures within our organization in order to move toward a "healthier community." I must emphasize that this second "Ah ha" experience built on learnings from the first visioning process in 1987. My shift in leadership style was a necessary foundation. Since we cannot anticipate nor predict future directions resulting from health care reform, visioning, creativity, and openness must be part of our daily processes.

• Conclusion

Leaders within health care organizations that are undergoing successful transformation typically experience new insights, awarenesses, and sensibilities regarding their own roles and responsibilities in the delivery of health care and those of others at all levels of the organization. Their experiences — usually described as "Ah ha" experiences — are often viewed in very positive terms as energizing and empowering, and they occur within the dynamics of visioning, values framework, or interactive planning and management to identify opportunities to fulfill the organizational mission.

References

1. *Bridging the Leadership Gap in Healthcare.* Executive Summary of a National Study Conducted by the Leadership Center of the Healthcare Forum. San Francisco: The Healthcare Forum, 1992.

2. Stein, M., and Hollwitz, J. *Psyche at Work: Workplace Applications of Jungian Analytical Psychology.* Wilmette, IL: Chiron Publications, 1992.

3. Storm, H. *Lighteningbolt.* New York City: Ballantine Books, 1994.

4. Rovin, S., and Ginsberg, L. *Managing Hospitals: Lessons from the Johnson & Johnson-Wharton Fellows Program in Management for Nurses.* San Francisco: Jossey-Bass, 1991.

Part Three

Facilitating Organizational Transformation

• Introduction to Part 3

The most important factor for the success of a reengineering effort is leadership. The entire complement of leadership skills are needed. Vision that reaches over the horizon is required or the organization will never begin reengineering. Communication that helps employees commit to something that does not even exist is a must. Abstract, nonlinear thinking is necessary to create real breakthroughs. Savvy is needed to cut through the inevitable political and personal barriers. Perseverance must be in large supply because the road is challenging and difficult and new.

> Reengineering the organization: an approach for discontinuous change, Tim Coan, *Quality Management in Health Care* 2(3):25, 1994

The new organization that honors the soul and the soul of the world will be . . . an organization that is as much concerned with what it serves as what it is, as much attentive to the greater world as the small world it has become. . . .

> *The Heart Aroused: Poetry and the Preservation of the Soul in Corporate America,* David Whyte

Once an organization chooses change and identifies opportunities for change through visioning, there often results a shift in relationships. The shift may be intrapersonal (a shift in the way individuals feel about themselves as they gain clearer goals, ideals, and values); interpersonal (a shift in relationships between staff members); and/or intraorganizational (a shift in relationships between different units and departments of the organization). It may begin to be experienced between health care institutions (interorganizational), or between institutions and segments of the community (intrasocietal).

In health care, rapid technological change, service diversification, and cost reduction activities are also forcing a dramatic shift in the relationships among hospitals; among hospitals and community care settings, social agencies, and businesses; among hospitals and educational institutions; and among hospitals and payers, unions, and policymakers. As a result, institutional alliances and partnerships are growing at an ever-increasing rate. With competing staff demands for resources, new technology, and new projects and services, fewer identical services are being offered by health care systems within the same marketplace. Although competition remains a force, health care organizations are working more collaboratively and interdependently to meet community needs through greater cooperation.[1]

Transformational leaders know that people are the organization's most valuable resource. Thus, such leaders encourage the work force to develop a natural rhythm between connectiveness and solitude and between independence and accountability. This approach results in increased productivity and a work force that is excited about and takes pride in its work, confident that each individual's contribution is important.[2-4] Through development of meaningful relationships, the organization's stakeholders learn the connection between personal input and desired outcomes for themselves, the institution, and the community. The cornerstone of this relationship-building process is trust. Trust exists within organizations that have defined their guiding principles and desired outcomes and whose leaders take responsibility for establishing a solid infrastructure that will support the change process and the new relationships.[5]

Part 3 consists of two chapters. Chapter 6, Building New Relationships, describes changes in relationships between people that occur as organizations establish interdisciplinary teams, use internal consultants, and develop education and training programs. Chapter 7, Supporting New Relationships, discusses the results of changes between units and departments in both organizational structure and culture as alliances are built in a collaborative and cocreative way for the improvement of community health status.

References

1. Bennis, W. *An Invented Life: Reflections on Leadership and Change.* Reading, MA: Addison-Wesley Publishing Co., 1993.

2. Covey, S. R. *The 7 Habits of Highly Effective People: Powerful Lessons in Personal Change.* New York City: Simon & Schuster, 1990.

3. Senge, P. M., Roberts, C., Ross, R. B., Smith, B. J., and Kleiner, A. *The Fifth Discipline Fieldbook: Strategies and Tools for Building a Learning Organization.* New York City: Doubleday, 1994.

4. Whyte, D. *The Heart Aroused: Poetry and the Preservation of the Soul in Corporate America.* New York City: Doubleday, 1994.

5. Rothstein, L. R. The empowerment effort that came undone. *Harvard Business Review* 73(1):20–31, Jan.–Feb. 1995.

Chapter 6

Building New Relationships

When we think of work, we only consider function, and so the soul elements are left to chance. Where there is no artfulness about life, there is weakening of the soul. It seems to me that the problem with modern manufacturing is not a lack of efficiency, it is loss of soul.

Care of the Soul, Thomas Moore

The vision of an ideal organizational transformation is based on relationships that transcend discipline and department boundaries to form connections between individuals, institutions, neighborhoods, communities, and societies. Although no well-established conceptual or institutional framework currently exists that demonstrates how to build relationships beyond traditional boundaries, many individuals and organizations are working on developing designs for such relationships. One such organization is The Foundation for Community Encouragement, Inc., a nonprofit foundation created by Scott Peck and others to teach the principles and values of community to individuals, groups, and organizations.[1] Another such organization is *Dia·Logos,* a nonprofit institute founded by William Isaacs with a team at the Organizational Learning Center of the Massachusetts Institute of Technology to promote generative learning and collaborative social action through dialogue.[2] True dialogue enables groups of people to transform their world by reshaping fundamental patterns of thought and action so as to harness the power of their collective intelligence. In *The Fifth Discipline Fieldbook,* Senge writes: "I cannot imagine building a learning organization without the practice of dialogue at its very center."[3] The new relational paradigm calls for interlocking concepts and models emphasizing the well-being of people and their relationship to their environment.[4,5] A fuller understanding of organizational life is achieved by developing a systems view that sees the organization as a living organism containing multiple integrated relationships, rather than as a machine.[6,7]

In *The Chalice and the Blade,* Eisler says that old roots of civilization were never eradicated as culture evolved.[8] Qualities such as love of life and nature, sharing rather than taking, caring for rather than oppressing, and power viewed as responsibility rather than domination have existed in civilizations throughout history. Although these qualities have been suppressed by social orders of dominance and hierarchies, they have not died out and appear in many organizations seeking beneficial transformation. Systems of rank are being replaced with partnerships that enhance each partner's capacity to think and work in synergistic ways for the common purpose. Transformational leaders build on the interpersonal relationships of people throughout the organization, and explore interactive and integrated options for future organizational structures.

This chapter describes guidelines that characterize the team process and strategies that various organizations are using to implement it. It also discusses new demands on the organization brought about by team process implementation in terms of training and structural changes.

• The Team Process

Today, there is significant pressure to manage smarter using fewer resources and yet still respond to external pressures from health care reform initiatives. One way to do this is to bring more people into the management process—that is, to create an environment in which teams of people from different levels of the organization can work together to improve service outcomes. Bob Siver, vice-president of managed care, All Children's Hospital, says:

> As a person responsible for designing managed care contracts, I am concerned with how to produce positive service outcomes that can reduce future utilization of inpatient care while reducing the overall cost of care, particularly if capitation is the next generation of payment. I am only one person with a defined set of knowledge; I need others to help me manage smarter. I need people with different views and ways of thinking, people who can ask questions—the "what ifs"—and I need people who think with a systems perspective, including thinking about the long-term future, not just today or two years from now.

As discussed in previous chapters, before an organization can effectively understand its destiny (identify what it should be doing), its leaders and staff must define a meaningful vision. Their next step is to identify desired outcomes and current reality. They then build consensus on selecting strategic interventions based on their vision and the opportunities for change they have identified. The nature of the intervention itself determines who should participate in its implementation by defining who will be affected by the outcomes. Usually disciplines from different departments come together as a team to begin implementation of the process.

For a team to function effectively, its members must utilize the concepts and tools associated with interactive planning, systems thinking, reengineering, and quality improvement learned through systematic institutionwide education programs initiated by top leadership and carried out to the unit-level and support areas. Ideally, top leadership champions what is taught, emulates desired behaviors, and consistently uses a common language. Key individuals are identified as facilitators and are trained by experts in quality management processes; and they in turn use "train the trainer" methods to ensure that people at every level of the organization are capable of operationalizing the improvement process. (The team facilitator role is discussed in a later section of this chapter.) Encouraging more people in more relational activities, such as team processes, instills vitality, not only to help the organization survive but also to establish it as an essential component of a community-based health care system.

Guidelines for Team Building

Many leaders, including quality improvement managers and organizational development specialists, express similar guidelines when they discuss the importance of relationships, particularly in terms of building and implementing teams to carry out innovative work to deliver improved value. Their aggregated guidelines include:

- Attention is paid to processes and systems in an effort to understand the organization's capability as a whole.
- Thoughts and ideas are encouraged from people throughout the organization; fear is replaced by recognition for their ideas with appropriate follow-up.
- Structure and direction are of utmost importance; people will be more productive if they know exactly what is expected and what is the desired outcome.
- Decisions are based on shared data, not guesswork; there is a focus on improving how work gets done, not simply on what is done.
- Strategic thinking is encouraged allowing for a creative intuitive process that involves synthesis of information and informal learnings to gain new insights.
- The focus is on value, using systems improvement processes; productivity and efficiencies will follow, giving a greater sustained return on investments.
- Trained people are needed to facilitate team processes to ensure a systematic approach; cross-functional teamwork is crucial for achieving speed of improvements and an organizational quality.

- Education is a necessary component for changing behavior; educational opportunities are most effective with an integrated strategic plan to eventually include everyone.
- Multiple relationships at all levels of the organization ensure communication and coordination of services.

These guidelines are illustrated in the model put into place by Hartford Hospital. The model shows an integrated management structure called collaborative management teams (CMTs) with quality partnerships.[9] (See figure 6-1.) In this model, an executive CMT, composed of the chief executive officer (CEO) and the vice-presidents for patient operations and medical affairs, integrates executive-level decisions with service-level CMTs such as cardiac services. The arrows from the ovals to the executive CMT are intended to

Figure 6-1. Hartford Hospital Management Structure

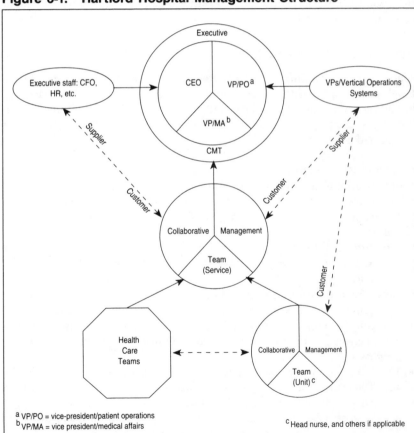

[a] VP/PO = vice-president/patient operations
[b] VP/MA = vice president/medical affairs

[c] Head nurse, and others if applicable

convey that vice-presidents responsible for functions such as finance and human resources continue to report directly to the CEO, whereas vice-presidents covering vertical operations systems with centralized support departments such as pharmacy and building services report to the chief operating officer (COO). The CMT levels below the executive level, including the unit level, are responsible for the customer–supplier relationships of their given services across inpatient and outpatient care settings. The customer–supplier relationship has evolved into a quality partnership designed to facilitate integration of vertical systems. The quality partners collaboratively define and determine desired patient care outcomes.

In *Collaboration in Health Care* by Stetler and Charns,[10] Rhonda Anderson, Al Herzog, and John Meehan describe how they came together from different paths to form the executive CMT at Hartford Hospital. Anderson had spent her professional life combining the functions of nursing practice with nursing leadership, Herzog was a clinician experienced in medical staff politics, and Meehan was a hospital administrator. What united these leaders was a shared vision of an innovative, patient-centered, hospitalwide delivery system that would continuously improve quality in a cost-effective manner. They described themselves as "competitive, energetic, goal-driven, and a self-starter." As they worked together, they strengthened their understanding of each other's talents and expertise, and formed a "nonconflictual management team" that served as a model for the rest of the institution on how to build trust and reach organizational outcomes despite dissimilarities in experience. One tool they used to clarify areas of role ambiguity was responsibility charting. This helped them to define tasks that were collaborative and those that were autonomous. Additionally, they all took the Meyers-Briggs Type Indicator (MBTI) test to learn about personal administrative styles and behaviors. "Understanding our various profiles helped us depersonalize our occasional differences during deep discussions," they agreed, although they stressed that to achieve a truly collaborative relationship, the MBTI should be combined with other leadership tools.

Strategies for Team Building

One of the first steps in assembling a team is to decide who should comprise its membership. William Manahan, medical director of quality assurance, indicates that at Immanuel-St. Joseph's Hospital "senior leadership began by selecting individuals to chair or cochair interdisciplinary teams who were interested in the topic or problem. We then selected individuals for the team who would be affected by the outcome and those that wanted to be on the team." Annette McBeth, vice-president, adds that:

> . . . people with known interpersonal skills, with innovative and creative potentials, those who attend to detail, and those who are decision

makers are useful characteristics to consider. People who are committed, goal oriented, enthusiastic, positive, and who have good technical skills also are excellent team members. Teams should be made up of a composite of people, since no one person brings all the talents needed to get the work done.

Stetler and Charns[11] advocate introducing a team member who is unfamiliar with a given project because, with appropriate training, this individual can be an excellent facilitator by asking "what if" questions or by saying "Help me understand what you are trying to accomplish." Other individuals recommended for team membership include people who are resistant to change, thinking about leaving the organization because they are dissatisfied, and informal leaders. For example, a respiratory therapist at MeritCare Health System said, "I was ready to leave; now three years later, after being on a work and role design team, I am excited and proud to be an associate of the hospital; I feel my opinion is important and I have a better understanding of our direction."

Sharon Lee, vice-president, patient care services, St. Luke's Regional Medical Center, suggests another element that might be considered in the team member selection process:

> Individual disciplines from clinical directors to service staff were involved in the interview and selection process for interdisciplinary teams. This process demonstrated the importance of having members selected by their own discipline or peer group. It also was an opportunity to learn about issues, problems, and biases which serve as a foundation to avert some problems in the future and strengthen interpersonal relationships.

An effective principle for beginning groups is to set ground rules at the outset. Jeannette Ullery of St. Luke's Regional Medical Center says, "Using agreed upon norms can quickly resolve conflicts or other issues. In my experience, interdisciplinary teams who identified norms and goals clearly at the beginning of their work made progress much easier. The struggles occurred with the groups when direction seemed vague or ambiguous, and they did not adhere to their ground rules." McBeth explains the team-building strategies used at Immanuel-St. Joseph's Hospital, including the establishment of ground rules:

> Useful strategies in fostering interdisciplinary teamwork include being attentive to everyone who is involved, identifying ground rules early in the group process, using these rules consistently throughout the life of the group, and agreeing on and mutually working toward a desired outcome. For example, we selected the orthopedic services as an area in which we wanted to reduce costs and improve quality of care. Our first

challenge was to identify the indicators for that service, using a team approach. The following indicators became the framework for our work together: patient and provider satisfaction, quality clinical outcomes, and cost reduction.

Next, we identified the key stakeholders — those people who would be affected by a change or who had an investment in the orthopedic service. Representative stakeholders were invited to the table to discuss how to impact the indicators. A project director and interdepartmental and interdisciplinary team members were identified. Because of the clinical components of this project, a clinician was selected as the project director. Time lines were spelled out and progress reports were expected at specified intervals. The team identified ground rules: Decisions were always to be in the best interest of patients and their families; quality of care resulting from the intervention must be impacted in a positive way; and cost reduction should result. A patient control group and subject group were identified and indicators of care were compared. The control patient group received their care in the traditional manner of the orthopedic service. The subject group care processes were outlined on a clinical pathway. A nurse case manager collaborated with the physician to manage the care across the in-hospital stay of the patient. As outcomes began to unfold and differences noted, the team became energized, realizing that their collective contributions were making a difference. People took ownership of the project. As one team member said, "We are designers or architects of an improved, cost-efficient service."

Open and honest communications were essential to the ability of this team to work together. As individuals struggled with a change of mind-set from "My department does this" to "We can do this together," it was apparent that communication expectations were needed. The team identified two key expectations: first, party communication — discussing issues with each other rather than taking them outside the group; and commitment to each other to become coworkers, each contributing value to the success of the whole project.

Additionally, accountability ground rules were outlined for the team and level of authority. As the team progressed in their work, their level of authority progressed. The senior manager coached the process for authority, assisting the team in their understanding of what the authority meant and preparing them for the next level. This gradual progression facilitated team empowerment while providing them a structure for why they do the work and assuming responsibility for outcomes. The levels identified are:

- Level 1: Gather information.
- Level 2: Gather information and make recommendations.
- Level 3: Gather information, make recommendations, and negotiate.

- Level 4: Exemplify the team norms and continue the process in other organizational activities — "Walk the talk."

At Tallahassee Memorial Regional Medical Center, the team process was based on planning boards at the unit and department levels. Brad Brown, vice-president, management information systems, describes his experience with overcoming barriers to team building:

> With the initiation of the information system (IS) planing boards, sessions were characterized by finger pointing, complaining, and emotional outbursts. Realizing that the IS staff was not going to be able to sort out their feelings — giving up the old to move to a new way of working — I shared my dilemma with the nurse executive. She suggested I give the staff an opportunity to grieve their losses by using a process that she found effective with her nurse managers. Taking her suggestion, I constructed a miniature coffin with "R.I.P." written on the side. It was placed in the center of the table. After the group shared their initial reaction, each member was asked to write on a sheet of blank paper the uncomfortable feelings or issues they had with another member of this group. They could name the person if they desired or just write their feelings or issues resulting from the experience. They were then instructed to fold the papers over and toss them into the coffin, serving notice, effective that very minute, that those issues were dead and buried, behind us and forgotten. The issues were not to enter into any further discussions. The session ended with a pledge from each person that should she or he have an issue with another person, the issue would be discussed face-to-face, exploring a mutual resolution. If a resolution was not achievable, the next step would be to involve me in the process. This became a group norm — first, to initiate conversation with each other. The overall response to this session was somewhat amazing. The group was soon laughing and joking. Some even offered to take the coffin out into the parking lot and burn it. The exercise helped to put in perspective the need for open and honest communications. While it has not been a complete cure for organizational communication barriers, I use it often as a lighthearted reminder of where we want to be. Since that session, the work of the planning boards are characterized by frank, open, and often lively conversations.
>
> The whole issue of creating teamness by bringing multiple disciplines together to create an interdisciplinary approach is paramount to an interactive planning environment. Everyone must feel they are part of the process and not token outsiders, if they are to contribute meaningfully. To achieve this environment, we instituted the following guidelines for interdisciplinary groups:

- *All are equal:* There is no ranking of individuals by status; organizational and functional titles are left at the door. (See the discussion below.)
- *"Tech-speak":* There is no tech-speak or systems terminology used during group discussions.
- *Automation:* There are no assumed answers; particularly, automation is not assumed to be the answer.
- *Opinions and ideas:* Everyone's opinions and ideas are valued, and all questions must be answered or given a reason why they cannot be answered.
- *Leadership:* The chair position rotates among team members, including grass-roots staff.
- *Overview of process:* Some members will be specifically trained in interactive planning; at a minimum, everyone is provided an overview of interactive planning.
- *Consensus:* Consensus building is the desirable method of decision making; although desirable, it is not mandatory.
- *"Dare to dream":* Everyone is encouraged to dream and use their imagination.

These guidelines are a framework, providing the team direction to determine its own balance of freedom and task orientation.

The first guideline above is somewhat controversial. Although many transformational leaders agree that leaving organizational titles at the door can encourage a spirit of equality, others question its value. For example, Norman Urmy, executive director, Vanderbilt University Hospital and The Vanderbilt Clinic, argues: "Are we trying to be something different than we are to create equality? For me, the key question is not whether one leaves his or her title at the door, but what is the strength of the person's expertise, and is that expertise respected?" Thomas Mroczkowski, vice-president/COO, Hackley Hospital, points out: "Titles can be left at the door when the work environment is conducive to open and honest communications. [However,] In an authoritarian-type structure, everyone on the team clearly knows where the power lies and what the consequences might be for an action that is unapproved or unsanctioned."

• Cross-Functional Teams

Cross-functional teams are a strategic tool for clinical and operational improvements. They are interdisciplinary in nature and represent more than one department or functional group. Project staff from Beth Israel Hospital indicate "interdisciplinary teams strengthen their relationships by developing a common vocabulary and instituting a common process for implementation of a desired outcome." The strategy of developing a notebook to record their process and identify group guidelines established consistency, and groups could learn from each others' work. McBeth and Manahan emphasize, "It is essential to provide the large amount of time needed for cross-functional teams to develop mature interpersonal relationships. As relationships grow, there is a higher level of trust and confidence displayed by staff, who become more independent and recognize the talents of individuals and what they can accomplish collectively. Their overall productivity increases, since energy is focused on what is best for the patient rather than negotiating what is best for each department." There is a caution, however, as pointed out by leaders who initiated cross-functional teams early in their change process. As teams become more interdependent, they seem self-sufficient and may loose some synergy with each other. Beth Israel Hospital, Abbott-Northwestern, and Providence Portland Medical Center operationalized cross-functional teams early in their restructuring process. They each experienced initial enthusiasm and enormous energy; however, a year or so into their restructuring effort things slowed down and the initial energy level dissipated. They each regrouped (revisioned) and put in place an organizational infrastructure integrating their clinical and operational systems improvements. That infrastructure is based on a strategically integrated educational program for all levels of management and staff, with interactive decision making and communications, and developmental standard or process charter. For Beth Israel, their notebook became the foundation of their developmental standard which is an essential component of their quality improvement program.

• Education and Team Building

Systematic educational activities are crucial to developing interdependent relationships. Activities such as idea borrowing occur naturally during team meetings, hallway conversations, and other organizational events. However, real education may not take place unless well-defined processes are in place to support informal and ongoing learning. According to Lee, "If appropriate education is not a part of the process, it makes it more difficult for people to shift out of old paradigms into new ways of looking at work and the systems involved in the process of work." However, hospital administrators often state that education and training are too expensive. The response among many transformational leaders is not whether the hospital can afford to provide its work force with education and training but, rather, can it afford not to. These leaders argue that if work teams are to be put in place, the work force must be taught how to take on its new responsibilities. Additionally, as Lloyd Smith, president/CEO, MeritCare Health System, points out: "There is significant value added to organizations when well-prepared work teams are put in place. The merge between MeritCare Hospital and the Clinic is a smoother process than anticipated because the hospital staff understands the importance of the new relationship, and they know how to integrate key activities."

Lack of work force training and education can result in a slowdown, if not a stoppage, in team process implementation. Organizations that did not initiate organizationwide education programs early in their restructuring found that teams lacked synergy and constancy in their work. These organizations had to stop their team process to develop and implement a specifically designed education program, including formal and "just-in-time" (JIT) training. Many brought in outside consultants to conduct a "train the trainer" or "coach the coacher" process. The goal of these organizations, and those that included education initially, is to be able to do their own educational activities, rather than rely on sustained consultant services. For example, Vanderbilt University Medical Center initially used a consultant to conduct a two-and-a-half-day leadership course for its managers. Recognizing the value of the course content and its potential results for improving clinical and operational decisions, the medical center trained its own staff to offer the program to all managers and project leaders. Judy Spinella, director/COO, describes the course as "a management philosophy that stresses the participation of all layers of staff in team decision making. It builds on our value of people and facilitates their informed involvement in operational and clinical management."

McBeth stresses the importance of top-level management commitment to education and training for the organization's work force as the organization implements the team process:

Executive commitment is essential for an institutionwide systematic, continuous education and training program for team development. This program ultimately should be a part of new employee orientation with periodic refreshers for everyone. To kick off team formation at Immanuel-St. Joseph's Hospital, key clinical and management leadership identified the first teams who were required to participate in a three-day education and training program on leadership empowerment of staff. An organization cannot be successful in developing them without committing resources to education and training. We also found after three years of experience, people want to attend development programs that no longer are required.

Organizations have used a number of guidebooks, workbooks, and fieldbooks as references for their training programs, including *The Team Handbook* by Scholtes,[12] *The Fifth Discipline Fieldbook* by Senge,[13] and several workbooks published by the American Hospital Association and others. Leaders, managers, and staff involved in quality management utilize concepts and tools from many experts and integrate information in the manner best suited for their organization. Computer networks, including Internet, CompuServe™, and HandsNet™, are additional resources.

Sometimes arguments against work force education and training have less to do with expense than with a basic skepticism about the team process itself. Mroczkowski explains:

> Skepticism about multiple people working together from different disciplines is understandable. In our traditional autocratic way of managing, we seldom asked employees what they thought. Now we are telling them that they are the ones who know best how to do their job, and they are the ones who can best design changes and improvements. An issue we continue to experience at Hackley Hospital is some employees feel what they are doing somehow is management work. When they are involved in some type of decision making, there is a question who should be doing that type of work—they or management.

Other leaders indicate similar concerns with no certain method of resolution. However, as mentioned previously, strengthened interpersonal relationships will improve staff trust and confidence that decision making is part of their responsibility. Systematic and strategic educational activities for management, together with unit staff, will help make the transition from top-down management to integrated partnerships between management and staff. Many senior leaders and other managers will have as much difficulty giving up decision making as staff have accepting it. When strategic attention and sensitivity are shown to perceived loss of decision-making authority, managers will be able to move forward, recognizing that their contribution is based on expertise and talent, not title or status.

• Training Demands on the Organization

Training people in the team process requires participation by people throughout the organization. The following sections examine the responsibilities of key positions in this process.

Team Leaders and Team Facilitators

In many cases, the team leader and team facilitator roles are filled by the same person; in others, they are handled by two different people. Generally, the *team leader* is someone who has a vested interest in the project and is respected by members of the group. He or she monitors the agenda and focuses on the desired outcome—in other words, on what is expected as a result of the team's effort. On the other hand, the *team facilitator* maintains objectivity, monitoring the flow of conversation and supporting the ability of everyone to contribute. Stetler advocates filling the team facilitator role with someone from outside the department—that is, someone who will not be affected by the outcome of the project.[14] An example of the types of individuals who might fill these roles may be found in a team involved in designing improvements for obstetric patients at Hartford Hospital. On that team, the clinical manager of the inpatient unit served as team leader and the chaplain served as team facilitator.

Both team leader and team facilitator are attentive to interpersonal relationships and team process structures. They often will use techniques such as role-play, stories, and quality improvement tools and processes to convey the message. Sometimes the team facilitator has responsibility for JIT training and the how of the process, and for coaching the team leader. When the roles are separate, it is important that their responsibilities be clearly defined. The team leader may be accountable for why the project is necessary and what outcomes are desired. Linda Fleury, human resource analyst, MeritCare Health System, describes the characteristics of an effective team leader as "the ability to listen, accept and give feedback, accept other ideas when they differ from the leader, allow everyone to contribute equally, and facilitate decision making." Often the team leader is the key to the team's effectiveness and success. The leader is a cheerleader, keeping everyone enthused and informal; a organizer, keeping to the agenda and task at hand; and a motivator, keeping everyone focused toward the end goal. As the objective outsider, the team facilitator may be timekeeper, negotiator, and sometimes peacemaker. Once a group takes ownership of their desired outcome, the facilitator's responsibility may become one of keeping the group focused and energized.

Hartford Hospital, Vanderbilt University Hospital, MeritCare Health System, and Harbor-UCLA Medical Center project staffs use a facilitator structure, and stress the importance of team facilitator and leader training. As mentioned in a previous section, an outside consultant often performs the initial training, with the intent of preparing internal people to carry out the training long-term. MeritCare Health System also developed an in-house team leader and facilitator program designed to improve communication at every level of the organization, recognizing that everyone in the organization is someone else's customer. It utilizes the talents of employees who exemplify effective communication skills, builds on their capabilities, and expands those behaviors through formal training and role modeling. Everyone in the hospital, from senior management to unit staff, has attended the training program. It is now a part of the employee orientation and refresher curriculum and is established as an element of continuing education.

Outside Consultants

Outside consultants bring objectivity and expertise to the team process by providing recommendations for tested methods. If, when, and how they are used often is determined by the basic characteristics of the organization. Dependent (hierarchical) organizations generally use consultants as centralized decision makers and directors of how to initiate a project or change, working in collaboration with senior management and the board of trusts in making decisions related to desired outcomes and how they are to be achieved. On the other hand, interdependent organizations tend to use consultants more as facilitators, mentors, and coaches. Sometimes the consultant's role shifts as the organization moves toward interdependency. For example, many SHNP leaders reported that they initially requested centralized use of consultants and then, after being exposed to the principles of interactive planning and management, systems thinking, and project management, changed the consultant function to that of team leader and process facilitator. Project funds requested for consultants were shifted to train the trainer programs, in which the consultant facilitated leaders and project staff in training key members. The organization then continued to maintain an ad hoc relationship with the consultant as one of its many external resources and a member of the organizational family. SHNP leaders agree that when a consultant is employed to facilitate change processes, he or she must be able to enhance the organization's vision, assist with strategic thinking, perceive the risk involved with change, and offer alternatives for resolution of difficulties. Additionally, once a consultant becomes a part of the team responsible for change, he or she is often aligned with a key person in the organization, such as a quality improvement or special projects director.

The selection process for a consultant can be as intensive as that for any key organizational leader. Sharon Lee and Jeanette Ullery, consortium project director, explain the selection process at St. Luke's Regional Medical Center:

> Consultants were utilized for their knowledge by providing information on specific issues or topics. They facilitated planning processes for specified areas, such as quality improvement, work and role redesign, and patient care delivery system innovations. We used people we knew from past contacts or had knowledge of from a demonstrated track record or [who were] referred by trusted colleagues. The candidate was interviewed, first by phone, and then brought on-site for interviews with executive leadership, project team members, and other people key to the change effort. During the interview, we determine the consultant's style—facilitator or director; comfort with making recommendations, rather than decisions; ability and interest to work with all levels of staff along with management; and their personal values.

Lee further explains the importance of finding a consultant who emulated the organization's philosophy of investing in people and building a patient-centered care system:

Recently the medical center contracted with a consultant to facilitate the last phase of implementation of transforming the organization from a traditional structure to a service design, including full implementation of interdisciplinary work teams. It was clarified up front that we did not require a design of our structure, rather we wanted assistance to focus on the potentials for our future, considering the turbulence in our environment. After telephone interviews with three candidates, we selected a consultant with experience in hospitals implementing patient-focused care. He was engaged to do an organizational assessment, offering external expert observations about our patient-centered process and what our potential issues might be. His findings would reflect the input from various work groups and other key people, rather than his own viewpoint. Work groups were given the expectation to be open and honest—we wanted to learn and improve. While he offered helpful suggestions, his value was that he was open to challenge and revision, providing us opportunities to deepen our understanding of what we wanted to achieve. He saved us time by facilitating our critical thinking and pushing us to pursue a clear action plan for implementation. As an outsider, he tactfully helped us cut through our political rhetoric which, in the past, has hindered forward movement. The organization also has a cadre of internal consultants.

At MeritCare Health System, Betty Sayers, group facilitator, and Ruth Hanson, project director, discuss working collaboratively as external (Sayers) and internal (Hanson) consultants. They emphasize the outside consultant's ability to bring objectivity and a fresh perspective to the team process. Following are the assumptions that underpinned the project design and helped formulate their working relationship:

- Insiders are incapable of accurately observing their own culture; an outsider consultant or facilitator is more able to "see" the culture.
- An external consultant, arriving with an open mind, is more likely to develop a rapport with the employees and engender the trust necessary for them to bring the hidden cultures to the surface.
- An external consultant is in the best position to safeguard confidentiality and sincerity because of his or her independent position.
- Stress arises when managers first see the dysfunctional norms of their work group in contrast to new, desirable norms. A skilled consultant, without a history in the organization, is needed to help managers work through such confronting members.
- Both individuals value honest, forthright communication, and agree early on to present differences and opinions to each other openly and immediately. They also agreed to admit their lack of knowledge by saying "I don't know." They would focus on the positive aspects,

especially the lessons learned that were acknowledged and freely shared, and role-model the benefits of positive feedback by giving it to individuals and groups, as well as to one another.
- Orientation of a consultant: Maximize the time and resources of consultants by providing them a thorough orientation or briefing on the organizational context, including barriers, active issues, key players, and the corporate language. Prepare the consultant before they arrive, so they will be aware of the "hot buttons," major concerns, cliques, and organizational biases of the participants.
- Consultants help organizations to: (1) discover their strengths and possibilities, (2) expand their view by bringing examples of best practices, and (3) save development resources by suggesting ideas and programs that have been effective in other businesses.

The consultant is challenged with integrating strategy, technological change, improvement processes, and humanistic aspects, including psychological and spiritual dimensions affecting the individual. Selection of the consultant becomes critical to the end product, particularly for an organization that has as one of its goals to create a resilient work force while maintaining cost efficiencies. Some of the knowledge and skills that may be important are familiarity with reward systems (discussed in chapter 7), work and role design, stress management, career planning and development, along with corporate strategies and continuous cost and quality improvement processes.[15,16] Although a consultant may not be experienced or expert in all areas, he or she should be able to implement or gain access to resources to meet needs as they present, maintaining a systems approach versus a compartmental approach to transformation.

Project Directors

Often the success of people working together is enhanced by a core project team, usually headed by a designated director or coordinator. Project directors are the internal consultants, or internal change agents. According to the project design team from Harbor-UCLA Medical Center, "They [project directors] are the initiator of motion which sets off other motions creating a ripple effect throughout the organization." Project directors bring projects to their colleagues in a way that is understandable, personal, and pertinent; and attempt to elicit their enthusiasm, commitment, and involvement. They represent the organization's leadership and promote its values; and part of their role is knowing where to get the expertise, resources, and means to get work done. Often they bridge the gap between unit-level staff and management, listening to both sides and offering options for strengthening relationships between the two levels. In the case of a consortium, the project director bridges the gap between hospitals and other facilities. In essence, project directors are the persistent force that keeps focus on the project's vision.

Ginger Malone, project director and internal consultant, Abbott-Northwestern Hospital, describes her role this way:

> I see myself as an influencer, a persuader, a processor of ideas, and a negotiator. I am also a juggler. With a project of the scope and size of the one at Abbott-Northwestern Hospital, I have a lot of balls in the air at any given time. My job is to keep all of them up, yet move in the right direction. Some days, I need to be a comedian, maintaining a sense of humor for myself and seeing the humor in situations that seem impossible until focus is achieve by everyone. When things get difficult, I rely on the guiding principle of the hospital: Patients are the reason why we exist and people are the reason why we excel.

The role changes as the project matures. Initially, the project director may feel as if he or she is the only believer, supporting an idea that is vague and amorphous. However, once the idea has meaning and people feel ownership of it, the project director role changes from one of urging and nurturing the team to focusing the team's energy in a defined direction, seeking the appropriate resources for continued productivity. Cheryl Stetler, project director, Hartford Hospital, describes the change in her role this way:

> As the project unfolds and becomes institutionalized, my role changes. Early on, I was overseeing the development of change structure, planning retreats, and overall project management; midway, I found myself involved in working through organizational change, helping others make the change happen — more hands-on and problem solving in nature; now I am a facilitator, coach, mentor, observer, and an organizational resource for restructuring and redesign initiatives.

Advocating the team's efforts throughout the change process, acknowledging and celebrating their accomplishments, and giving credit to the team also are important. Susan Beck, project director, University Hospital/University of Utah, adds:

> Tenacity is critical to the role. It is not easy to make things happen, especially during the early stages. One day people may say they are committed, the next they have reasons why they are not. It is like a roller coaster until there is maturity and buy-in deepens.

The project directors at Harbor-UCLA Medical Center work together as co-principal investigators (PIs). Peggy Nazarey, director of nursing; Maryalice Jordan-Marsh, research division director of nursing; Paula Siler, professional practice division director of nursing; and Susan Goldsmith, coordinator and organizational development specialist, describe their team role as follows:

> As PIs, we are the leaders of the organizational change taking place at the medical center. We provide a context for and oversight of the change process and related idea design. We act as interval consultants and serve as historians. As a team, we are responsible for project operations and take leadership in how the change process unfolds, moving from paper to practice. As we carry out collaborative efforts, we have found the principles of organizational development to be critical.
>
> We purposefully assembled a team that had multiple skills and divergent perspectives and deliberately included individuals with no nursing experience and, in one case, no health care experience. We combined dedicated project staff and people with other responsibilities who committed a portion of their time. We found this to be an essential combination, since each member of the team had a special niche and different ties to the larger organization.
>
> As a team, we developed an organizational design model as a catalyst for change. To activate this model in our setting, we used a behind-the-scenes agenda-setting technique. This technique involves looking ahead, as in interactive, backwards planning (a principle of interactive planning and management) and then constructing time lines from that planning. The length of the time line varies with the project at hand—a month, a year, or more. Meetings are scheduled with an agenda identifying outcomes and minutes allotted per topic. The team reflects on possible pitfalls and serendipitous side effects and plans meeting processes to minimize problems and maximize benefits. We scrutinize the potential in existing resources and plan for integration of project activities with priorities of other campus groups.
>
> After meetings, we process what happened and revise, revise, revise. Even our own meetings come under scrutiny. We see what happens and unfolds in our group as a potential microcosm of the organization. We learn from each other and work to have our project groups do the same. Our intent is to build from recognition and appreciation of our different strengths, talents, and styles. We capitalize on our successes, promoting a sense of ownership among the project director team members for specific activities and a joint accountability for the whole. We often pair or break into small groups to manage these activities and set up similar pairings for groups in our project structure. Our key project groups all have co-leaders from different departments.
>
> We support each other in risk taking and capitalize on our successes. We encourage quiet venting of frustrations and public celebrations of what works. We continually explore how to have unity without

compromising our diversity. As we carry our work into the larger organization, we have sometimes had delays as each group grows accustomed to this approach to agenda setting, paring, and valuing of diversity. However, overall, as the culture and organizational change model catches on, we feel we are on the right track.

Managers

Managers and unit staff need to be trained in the team-building process together. In the early days of team building, some institutions trained only senior leaders and those unit staff who were members of interdisciplinary teams, rather than including middle and line managers. Sometimes this created a power struggle between line managers who were not included in the training program and their unit staff members who were. Occasionally, this resulted in a staff member not being released from operational work to participate in the team process. However, drawing middle and line managers into the process and providing them an overview of the training usually produces a change of attitude. Once they are comfortable, managers may express concerns about their perceived loss of authority and, indeed, their fear of job loss. As managers become familiar with the team process, they understand that, as teams become more self-reliant and self-directed, their role will change from one of supervising staff within boundaries to one of managing interactions and functions across boundaries. In *Leadership Is,*[17] Owen discusses the differences between traditional management and true leadership by using the concept of "open space," where employees are left free to do their work and manifest "spirit" while the leader attends to the boundaries. He writes: "The function of leadership is to grow structure, not impose it . . . leadership grows appropriate structure by honoring the Open Space, maintaining the boundaries, and encouraging Spirit to find its own form . . . leadership invokes and invites Spirit to lay down new footprints. Management paves the path, keeps the troops on schedule, and on the road."

When managers accept both teaching and learning roles, their commitment to the team process and their respect for the team's work builds goodwill and enthusiasm. Fleury summarizes:

As team processes take on operational importance, we [managers] have to be sensitive to the fact the unit-level employees have their unit work as well as their teamwork. Managers need to be involved in the balancing of those responsibilities, and they need to understand how the involvement of staff may affect their management functions.

Physicians

Physician involvement in the team process raises a unique set of issues, primarily because the role of the physician in the hospital is unique. Although physicians tend to agree that teamwork is vitally important, they recognize that sometimes there are barriers to their participation. William Manahan, medical director of quality assurance, Immanuel-St. Joseph's Hospital; Stephen Entman, professor/vice-chair, obstetrics and gynecology, Vanderbilt University Hospital; and Richard Lindsay, head, Division of Geriatric Medicine, School of Medicine, University of Virginia, explain:

> Physicians benefit from one-to-one contacts with people they respect and work with side by side in the clinical area. Informal hallway conversations between caregivers can be very effective when in the early stages of changing practice patterns, such as through the development of clinical pathways. Physicians may feel, rightly or wrongly, they have more insight into clinical issues, therefore find it difficult to participate in team meetings to discuss such issues. It is extremely hard for them to take time to sit comfortably at a meeting and truly be a part of the team, not just physically but emotionally and mentally. This may be one of the largest barriers for physicians becoming team players. Teamwork requires collaboration, and collaboration requires process, and process requires sitting down and spending time with each other discussing and talking. The intensity and acuity of patient care often takes the physician away or prevents concentration on the discussion. Physicians need to understand what is in it for them and their patients before they can commit to a process. Once they get hooked on what can improve and how the effort matches the needs of health reform, they will be enthusiastic.

These physicians also advocate early involvement of attending physicians with medical students and residents in teaching institutions in order to prepare future caregivers for collaborative processes and different working relationships.

• Structural Demands on the Organization

Because collaborative ventures between disciplines, between departments, and between inpatient and outpatient care settings can be an outgrowth of interdisciplinary teamwork, these ventures often make new procedural demands on the organization. Managers and employees involved in these relationships must be able to vary some of their traditional procedures, particularly communication systems.

Communication Systems

Organizations operationalizing collaborative ventures usually move from a vertical (up-and-down) system of communication to one that is both horizontal and vertical, allowing communication to move in all directions — in- and outside the hospital walls. The degree to which an organization changes its communication system depends on the potential value of the relationships that evolve and the desired outcome that can be achieved. For example, an organization may place a high value on relationships resulting from teamwork and staff empowerment, but also must consider demands of time, energy, and resources. The definition of *value* given in chapter 1 bears repeating here: improved quality, better service, and lower cost. Value helps evaluate what is desirable in any possible alternatives and the consequences of those alternatives. The transformational organization seeks to build collaborative behaviors throughout the institution or health care system through congruency in organizational structure, processes, and management style.

However, there are times when the executive leaders and boards of trustees must make decisions they deem to be in the best interest of the organization — for example, mergers between hospitals or hospitals and clinics, or even in buy-out and hospital closure. Those organizations demonstrating interdependent behaviors will make tough decisions with the well-being of everyone in mind, including the community they serve. Their top-level leaders will be sensitive to the human aspects of their decision making. In such situations, employees may not like the outcome but will have the information they need to understand why the decision was made and will be given opportunities to pursue other options. Those organizations demonstrating dependent behaviors may not show the same degree of sensitivity to their employees' well-being. Their decision making may be top-down with little thought given to providing explanations for their actions to either their employees or the community they serve.

Senior-level management and boards of trustees need to empower up front all individuals within the organization who will be affected by a given change. The organization will benefit if those individuals are empowered to design the process, implement the mutually agreed-upon intervention, and evaluate the effectiveness of the outcome through team processes. Executive leaders are encouraged to remain in the background, facilitating, mentoring, and coaching the process toward the desired outcome. Once a team is empowered appropriately, accountability can shift from individuals or departments to teams. Providing everyone the necessary tools and structure is essential to building an empowered, self-reliant work force. A defined structure and clear expectations of what is desired are critical components, along with developing interpersonal relationships and integration of the operational systems as part of the process.

Decision-Making Procedures

Until an organization can institutionalize an integrated structure, it often leaves in place parallel structures for decision making. One structure includes the existing chain of command and the other demonstrates an integrated structure for innovative activities such as quality improvement, cost reductions, and work and role design. This presents a dilemma. With two structures in place, it is difficult to move the team process from the innovation stage to the implementation and follow-through stages. There may be commitment from senior-level leadership for a pilot or demonstration, but when it comes to a change institutionwide, the traditional needs of departments and disciplines sometimes supersede those of the project, particularly if cost reduction is a major pressure. Cost reduction activities force many organizations into short-term thinking and departmental strategies, such as downsizing.

However, organizations that use integrated structures for critical decision making such as cost reduction find that employees throughout the organization feel responsibility for the organization as an entity. For example, a small rural hospital in south central Minnesota used its integrated structure to involve everyone in deciding the hospital's fate. The staff, including nursing, housekeeping, laundry, dietary, and others, along with administration and the board of directors, focused their energy on what type of service their community needed and how they could better meet those needs. They held open forums in the community to gather information, involving physicians and hospital leaders from a larger neighboring community to help them identify strategies. The result was that the hospital has been kept open, but is now under reconfiguration to become an outpatient service with a few remaining inpatient beds for limited-stay patients. The hospital has secured commitment from local primary care physicians and specialty physicians within the larger neighboring community to provide dedicated time to the outpatient service. In this scenario, hospital administration collaborated with everyone (staff and community), sought their involvement, and believed in what they collectively could contribute to improving the health care system in the community. Although this process resulted in a reduction in staff, strategies were outlined to allow for the dignity and well-being of the released work force. As one employee observed: "This hospital and the community will never be the same. We know why we need each other and how to work together for our common interest. We are no longer in competition; we are collaborators for what is best for all players."

• Conclusion

Teamwork and interpersonal relationships form the nucleus of actualizing the vision of organizational transformation. These relationships often result in the formation of true community by the essential stakeholders, who talk and think together in ways that inspire collaborative and coordinated action. The team process is an effective operational tool used to bridge the gap between defining and realizing opportunities established by visioning and framing values.

References and Notes

1. For more information, contact: The Foundation for Community Encouragement, Inc., 109 Danbury Road, Suite 8, Ridgefield, CT 06877 (203/431-9484).

2. For more information, contact; *Dia·Logos,* P.O. Box 42-1149, Cambridge, MA 02142 (617/576-7986).

3. Senge, P. M., Roberts, C., Ross, R. B., Smith, B.J., and Kleiner, A. *The Fifth Discipline Fieldbook: Strategies and Tools for Building a Learning Organization.* New York City: Doubleday, 1994.

4. Capra, F. *The Turning Point: Science, Society, and the Rising Culture.* New York City: Bantam Books, 1982.

5. Wheatley, M. J. *Leadership and the New Science: Learning about Organization from an Orderly Universe.* San Francisco: Berrett-Koehler, 1992.

6. Ackoff, R. L. *Creating the Corporate Future.* New York City: John Wiley and Sons, 1981.

7. Senge, P. M. *The Fifth Discipline: The Art and Practice of the Learning Organization.* New York City: Doubleday, 1990.

8. Eisler, R. *The Chalice and The Blade: Our History, Our Future.* San Francisco: Harper and Row, 1988.

9. Stetler, C. B., and Charns, M. P. *Collaboration in Health Care: Hartford Hospital's Experience in Changing Management and Practice.* Chicago: American Hospital Publishing, 1995.

10. Stetler and Charns.

11. Stetler and Charns, p. 22.

12. Scholtes, P. R. *The Team Handbook.* Madison, WI: Joiner Associates, 1992.

13. Senge, Roberts, Ross, Smith, and Kleiner.

14. Stetler and Charns.

15. Cummings, T. G., and Worley, C. G. *Organization Development and Change.* 5th ed. St. Paul: West Publishing Co., 1993.

16. Gibson, J. L., Ivancevich, J. M., and Donnelly, J. H., Jr. *Organizations, Behavior, Structure, Process.* 8th ed. Burr Ridge, IL: Richard D. Irwin, Inc., 1994.

17. Owen, H. *Leadership Is.* Potomac, MD: Abbott Publishing, 1990.

Chapter 7

Supporting the New Relationships

> Excellence in management will be achieved through an organizational culture of civility routinely utilizing the mode of community. Such organizations will be so dramatically successful, that is, cost effective, that their sister institutions—no matter how initially threatened—will flock to discover their secret and imitate them. . . . If the top managers of a company are the kinds of people who want community, then they can have it.
>
> *A World Waiting to Be Born: Civility Rediscovered,* M. Scott Peck

It is not enough to build new relationships, leadership also must adjust organizational culture to support them once they are in place. It must be prepared to overcome inevitable tension and resistance to change, create structures that will enable the change to operate smoothly and effectively, develop an assessment process to evaluate how the change is working, and be prepared to support the new behaviors in the desired culture through recognition and reward programs.

This chapter discusses how organizations deal with encouraging and rewarding new behaviors brought about by the change process. It also describes different structural models that will facilitate the change process.

• Supporting the Culture of Change

As mentioned in chapter 6, until an organization institutionalizes an integrated structure, it often supports parallel structures: one for chain-of-command decision making and one for performing innovative activities such as quality improvement. In addition to making it difficult to implement innovations, parallel structures frequently produce tension. For example, relationships between staff at different levels of the organization and across departments and disciplines can become strained as individuals and departments compete for funds or disagree over who has authority and accountability for decision making. Tension is an inevitable part of change; and despite the discomfort that it generally causes, it can be good for the organization because it generates creative energy. In fact, organizations undergoing transformational processes often value tension. Although tension usually is equated with conflict, transformational leaders understand that conflict in human affairs can be healthy and normal. Thus, they deal with conflict openly through respectful discussion and clarification, creating a forum in which opportunities for new relationships and potentialities for improvement can be explored. In *A World Waiting to Be Born,* Peck writes that dealing with conflict in this manner is the essence of civility and that "conflict is only uncivil when it is either hidden or unnecessarily blown out of proportion."[1]

Although there is no one method for handling organizational tension, a systematic, collaborative, and constant process (such as the value framework process or interactive planning and management process described in chapter 4) used over time usually will result in lessening tension between the parallel structures. In his work on institutionalizing transformations, Gilmore indicates that change efforts have a life cycle—beginning, mid-life, and ending. The beginning is characterized by enthusiasm for the potential of the desired outcome; in mid-life, progress slows, tension builds, and reality takes over; and the ending is the time to reflect, consolidate insights, revise, and celebrate.[2,3] At each stage of the life cycle, attention to humanistic elements and organizational values is as important as the operational process.

Tension and disappointment always result when old structures are being pushed to establish new ones. Wendy Baker, formerly of the Center for Patient Care Innovation (CPCI), Vanderbilt University Hospital and Clinic, describes the personal abilities that were useful to her in dealing with the tensions and conflicts that arose as her role changed:

> The center is a place where ideas blossom and people have the opportunity to unlock the organization's potentials by using their wisdom, talents, and skills. My role is to provide leadership through facilitation and collaboration, planning and developing innovations for the improvement of patient care services. The following abilities where useful to me as my role evolved from a staff approach (carrying out the details of scheduling, reporting, and doing) to a facilitator and mentor (teaching and coaching others as an internal consultant):
>
> - Be comfortable working through others to establish and move toward the vision of the organization

- Use strategic thinking to see the big picture and be willing to let others carry out the details, coaching them along the way, especially helping them overcome organizational hurdles
- Use active listening to understand where the threads of individual and organizational vision come together
- Work with staff effectively and comfortably from many levels of the organization and across disciplines
- See "red flags" in the change process
- Raise issues others may not want to hear
- Use facilitator skills and techniques for meetings and projects
- Demonstrate a working knowledge of the core management and improvement processes of the organization
- Conduct a critical stakeholder analysis and have the patience to spend the time getting agreement from a diverse group
- Use effective project management skills, including follow-through techniques
- Understand the politics and priorities of the organization
- Be knowledgeable and facilitate a practical and responsive evaluation process

The value of the center is as an internal consulting agency, providing expertise to faculty and staff on meeting planning; project facilitation; collaborative care designs, including case management and clinical pathways; clinical and operational process improvements; work and role redesign; and evaluation. CPCI experienced tensions and conflicts similar to an outside consultant. In the developmental and early implementation stage, there was a tendency to dominate dedicated staff time with projects generated by executive management. It was necessary to create a balance between the priorities of executive leadership and the needs as perceived by lower-level staff. Now the organization knows how to deal with them; there is a collaborative structure in place at the unit and department level that allows for shared leadership and participation by all levels of staff. The CPCI structure is based on the principles of interactive planning and circular organization work of Russell Ackoff.

Anne Payne, associate dean/chair of the department of nursing, Boise State University, talks of the difficulties in overcoming tension and conflict caused by the traditional boundaries between service and education:

Those barriers had to be understood and painfully worked through before trust, and finally acceptance, could take place. The whole department now embraces our vision, including it as a written part of our strategic plan. The vision states education and service can blend, bond, and collaborate to capitalize on one another's strengths. We can work with our practice partners to teach more effectively and efficiently. We can do more to lend our expertise to practice settings and thereby cross-fertilize and decrease institution educational costs. We have a new way of partnering now—the teaching partnership concept.

We also are piloting a challenging experiment that has the potential to change the socialization of students in nursing, radiological sciences, and respiratory therapy. The beginning step is a multidisciplinary course that will teach basic patient care assessments and universal patient care skills. The course will be followed with other activities or courses that will bring the students together so they can learn to think and intervene as a team, not just as a discipline. The vision is limited to a few nursing faculty. Through dialogue and other collaborative processes, this vision will be endorsed by the entire department and maybe even by the university as a whole. The biggest challenge for faculty colleagues is to overcome the expected resistance such as threat to job and autonomy. The faculty, myself included, are learning strategies to "unfreeze" the paranoia and move to a new collaborative relationship. If a leader has a deep-seated need for acknowledgment, recognition, or power, I would recommend not initiating a process of this nature. The leaders should be able to stand back and take pride, not credit, in the accomplishment of colleagues as they strive together toward a shared vision. Most of all, leadership must remember that the vision is an abstraction by its very nature. The operationalization of that vision is a rich process of human creativity and enthusiasm. The reward is in seeing the unfolding and final product of attaining the vision, not the applause or accolades of an audience. There was pain and disappointment during the change in thinking, behavior, and relationships. However, the important thing about the conflict, pain, and struggle is that they did not overcome or obstruct our work together. In many ways, they became a source of energy to move forward, because we knew change was needed and it was the right thing to do.

• Changing Structures to Support Organizational Transformation

Organizations experiencing change in management and operational structures that support clinical and operational processes often have different end points. Some health care organizations (for example, MeritCare Health System, Fargo, North Dakota; Tallahassee Memorial Medical Center, Tallahassee, Florida; and District of Columbia General Hospital, Washington, DC) took an institutionwide approach to transformation. All were successful after more than five years of planning, development, implementation, and revisioning. During that time, all experienced the gamut of emotional responses to change—resistance and acceptance, tension/conflict and creative energy, disappointment and satisfaction—as they moved toward demonstrating cost-efficient and high-quality care outcomes.

Some organizations promote interplay between vertical integration (improvement or innovation from one level of the organization to the other) and horizontal integration (improvement or innovation across departments and disciplines at the same level); others concentrate initially on making changes either horizontally or vertically. For example, Hartford Hospital, in Hartford, Connecticut, initiated horizontal integration using collaborative management teams as the foundation for its change in management structure.[4] (See chapter 6.) A year or more into the change process, the hospital recognized the value of making changes horizontally to improve operational systems throughout the organization. On the other hand, University Hospitals of Cleveland, in Cleveland; Mercy Hospital and Medical Center, in Chicago; and University Hospitals/Pennsylvania State University, The Milton S. Hershey Medical Center, in Hershey, Pennsylvania, were successful in achieving their desired outcomes for horizontal integration and eventually moved to include aspects of vertical integration. In some cases, particularly the latter two, the horizontal improvement structure quickly encouraged the need for vertical changes. In both these institutions, the intent was to create a fundamental change in the delivery of patient care services. Processes were initiated at the unit level and eventually spread to the department level and throughout the organization.

University Hospitals of Cleveland's demonstrated integration by developing a collaborative model of care delivery. The model is based on the principles of case management, which is a needs–response approach to patient care. The model emphasizes the collaboration of multiple disciplines across departments and care settings. The focus of the collaboration is to coordinate health care services to high risk populations. The model, also is horizontally integrated across four community hospitals involved in an informal network hospitals implemented a common standard of collaborative care for the stroke population. Now nurses, physicians, and other health professionals work together in each of the hospitals to ensure similar patient care outcomes throughout the network. Patient care outcomes include length of stay, cost of service, patient satisfaction, and quality indicators such as readmission, medication error rates, and infection rates.

Mercy Hospital and Medical Center implemented horizontal integration through collaborative management groups (CMGs), which are described later in this chapter. These groups bring physicians and nurses together to coordinate the care of specific patient populations, such as cardiac and neurology patients, across care settings. As the groups evolved, members recognized the need to design and implement systems operation improvements. They joined other departments and disciplines to form cross-functional teams (cross department) to enhance the utilization of labor and technological and supply resources as they provide services to patients and their families. CMGs and cross-functional teams gradually influenced a participative decision making structure between senior level and unit level managers. The structure allows staff from the unit level to directly participate in strategic decisions that affect improvements for patient services organizationwide.

University Hospitals/Pennsylvania State's circular design model, discussed later in this chapter, initially started as a horizontal integration across clinical departments. It has evolved to a model that facilitates relationships between clinical and operational departments including an integration of the decision-making structures from the executive level to the unit level.

According to the experiences of SHNP leaders, both integrations are necessary for fundamental cultural change. It is clear that vertical integration ultimately could not affect the institution unless it was complemented by horizontal integration. Organizations find it more difficult to effect vertical integration than horizontal integration, primarily because vertical change deals more with actual management models and styles — authoritarian to participatory. Changing management styles raises issues of power, authority, and spheres of control as opposed to issues of influence, competency, and empowerment. Many of the behaviors and thinking associated with the authoritarian structure are so ingrained in leadership that changing them takes a great deal of time and understanding, as well as a rationale that supports leadership's personal belief and commitment to change.

However, whether the organization starts the process with horizontal or vertical integration, or both simultaneously, seems to depend on its readiness for change; the ability of its people to effect change; and the strength of its leadership's commitment to change. Overall, integration processes have prepared institutions for the cost reduction initiatives and reimbursement alternatives resulting from health care reform. Connie Murphy, director, patient care project, Mercy Hospital and Medical Center, explains:

> The overall goal is to transform the organization from patient centered, but department driven, to one which is patient driven. *Patient driven* is defined as "an organization in which the employee is empowered to respond to the individual needs of the patient, instead of the routine of the system." To accomplish this goal, three objectives were identified to guide our work: (1) develop meaning, practice, and a philosophy of patient driven by providing the employee a clear vision of patient care and their own responsibility; (2) implement a system of patient care delivery in which each patient is a participating mer..Jer of a collaborative care management team consisting of a primary physician, primary and associate nurses, and appropriate members of the mulitdisciplines; and (3) restructure the Mercy organization which supports timely decision making on the patient's behalf by the collaborative

management model. The collaborative management model, which is the foundation of the project, is an exclusive relationship between the patient and a care team. The model provides for the integration of services across the continuum, including the physician's office, inpatient care, outpatient, and wellness care. The model has influenced collaborative relationships between care providers and leadership, resulting in physician and nurse participation in strategic decision-making processes. The supporting management structure for the collaborative model includes a formal institutional mechanism for patient care innovations and improvements.

Circular Design Model

Guided by the principles of Ackoff's model of circular organizations,[5] University Hospital/Pennsylvania State University, The Milton S. Hershey Medical Center, implemented a collaborative management model called HORIZONS: Partnerships in Patient Care, which is designed to facilitate relationships between clinical and operational systems and eventually result in both horizontal and vertical integration. The intent of the model is to address systemwide problems in order to improve patient care, enhance the quality of work life, and create cost efficiencies.[6] Figure 7-1 depicts this circular organization model. In a circular organization, planning and decision making are driven by multidisciplinary, multilevel boards as described by Alan Barstow in chapter 4. The Medical Center has three levels of boards: eight service boards (clinical specialty), three unit boards (geographic location), and the project steering

Figure 7-1. Model of the Circular Organization

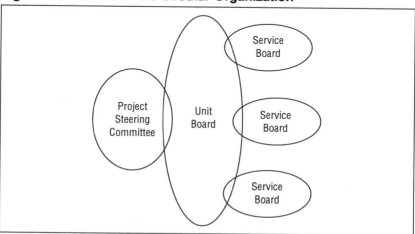

Source: HORIZON's Partnership in Patient Care, University Hospitals/Pennsylvania State, The Milton S. Hershey Medical Center, Hershey, Pennsylvania.

committee that provides guidance for the overall HORIZONS project. Membership on these three levels of boards overlaps—the chairs of the individual service boards are also members of their respective unit boards, and the chairs of the unit boards are committee members of the project steering committee.[7] The boards are empowered, within their department or service, to recommend and implement clinical and system improvements. For example, the pediatric service board resolved a laboratory specimen issue that was delaying the discharge time of a specific group of pediatric patients. The board included all stakeholders who could affect the change including pediatric nurses and physicians, admission staff, and clinical laboratory staff. Identifying the desired outcome of a decreased length of stay for the group of pediatric patients, the stakeholders selected the intervention of addressing the timely response of reporting laboratory results.

At the same time that the institution initiated the HORIZONS structure, it introduced a continuous quality improvement (CQI) process, later followed by a cost-reduction process. The HORIZONS structure focuses on improvements of clinical systems (the services provided directly to the patient by care providers (physicians, nurses, and other professionals). The CQI process addresses operational systems improvements (systems providing support functions such as medical supplies, pharmacy, and radiology). In contrast, cost-reduction strategies address the utilization of resources including labor, technology, and supplies. All three initiatives use principles of systems thinking, quality improvement, and interactive planning. However, each of the initiatives has a different decision-making structure. HORIZONS was led by nursing administration and the other two are led by operations administrators. Recognizing that, at times, these initiatives duplicate resources and involve many of the same people, the hospital integrated the three initiatives into a unified effort organizationwide. Joan Lartin-Drake, project director for HORIZONS, suggests the following guidelines for achieving the integration:

- Share ownership with operations leadership and staff identifying their accountability and responsibility
- Provide opportunities for affected stakeholders to talk together, and value these opportunities
- Change from "power over" to "power to and with"
- Learn to respect the difference facilitating a change from a conflict-avoidance culture to one that views conflict as creative energy
- Pace change according to the organization's ability to deal with it
- Define empowerment and provide a structure for all participating in the process
- Provide safety for risk taking and trust building
- Provide opportunities to share early learnings and successes
- Revision, revision, and revision

Shared Governance Model

Another structural model, also circular in design, is the partnership or shared governance model. In this model, members of a consortium combine their efforts to improve health care delivery within a specific region by sharing resources, leadership development, coordinated action, and innovative work groups. Its structure is that of an executive committee at the decision-making core, surrounded by associated standing committees. An example of this model is case-studied in chapter 12. Called Health BOND (Building Opportunities and New Directions) and formed for the purposes of SHNP, it is a voluntary, noncontractural consortium located in south central Minnesota and consisting of three hospitals—Immanuel-St. Joseph's Hospital, Arlington Municipal Hospital, and Waseca Area Memorial Hospital—and two educational institutions—Mankato State University and South Central Technical College.

Two similar governance structures designed to promote integrated clinical services between rural and urban hospitals and other community care settings are the Rural Connection in Idaho, which includes rural and urban hospitals (St. Luke's Regional Medical Center and Idaho Elk's Rehabilitation Hospital, in Boise; McCall Memorial Hospital, in McCall; Walter Knox Memorial Hospital, in Emmett; Wood River Medical Center, in Hailey and Sun Valley; and Holy Rosary Medical Center, in Ontario, Oregon) and Boise State University; and the Montana Consortium, which includes six community hospitals (St. Vincent Hospital and Medical Center, in Billings; Columbus Hospital, in Great Falls; Community Memorial Hospital, in Sidney; Frances Mahon Deaconess Hospital, in Glasgow; St. Joseph Hospital, in Polson; and St. Patrick Hospital, in Missoula). The Montana Consortium promotes linkages and relationships among hospitals by establishing a shared educational curriculum for hospital members desiring to restructure their environments operationally and clinically. The curriculum uses the interactive planning and management process, systems thinking, and project management and evaluation principles. Each of these consortia is strengthening its community development efforts as it designs strategies to affect the community's health status. Community-focused strategies include teenage pregnancy prevention programs, parenting classes, classes for caregivers of elderly family members, nutrition classes, and screening programs. Efforts emphasize the involvement of community leaders, families, and other residents.

Additionally, some leaders, such as Lynne Mattison, consortium director for Montana, are pursuing Creating Healthier Communities fellowships for health care leaders with The Healthcare Forum: Leadership Strategies for Healthcare, in San Francisco. The fellowship is designed to provide applied learning experiences to cultivate the transformational leadership necessary to cooperatively create solutions to a community's health needs. One of its end goals is to create community partnerships for improved community health status. This will be achieved in part through a self-directed action research project designed to enhance the health status of the individual fellow's immediate community.

• Determining an Appropriate Assessment Design and Process

Determining an appropriate assessment design and process that can be used to demonstrate the effectiveness of outcomes resulting from a transformational process and the work of transformational leaders remains an enigma. However, transformational leaders agree that an evaluation cannot be a pure experimental design, meaning that it has to allow for interpretation of and adaptability to whatever is being changed due to the dynamic—and sometimes chaotic—nature of change. The rigor of the assessment design is not only to demonstrate a cause-effect finding (program effectiveness) but also to validate that the finding is meaningful. That is, a good evaluation will try to explain why a program has been effective and also will be grounded in practical meaning for the users of the end product. For example, one aspect of a cardiac unit that is grounded in patient-centeredness is the goal of providing each patient with the opportunity to select from a daily menu of items, which meet medical limitations (that is, salt or volume restriction) but still allow options for specialty dishes that would satisfy, even delight, multiple cultural or ethnic desires. A good evaluation would measure success, such as providing kosher foods preferred by a Jewish patient. Whatever the assessment method, quasi-experimental, action or learning research, or responsive evaluation, it should be grounded in evaluation fundamentals using pragmatic language. SHNP found it practical to use a utilization-focused design, which is a process for making a decision about the usefulness of the intervention (focus) and content of the evaluation.[8] The content is determined through the collaborative interactions of affected stakeholders (caregivers, managers, executive leaders, and, as appropriate, patients and their families, trustees, educators, and payers) who will determine an intervention's effectiveness using the assessment results. The evaluation is geared to the interest, needs, and capabilities of the people involved. It provides them the opportunity to raise questions such as, "What difference does that information or intervention make?" and "What would you do if you had an answer to that question?"

John Romas, J.A.R. and Associates, and Annette McBeth, vice-president, Immanuel-St. Joseph's Hospital, discuss the importance of focusing on a consistent evaluation model:

In the past, we based our evaluation on competitive models, i.e., numbers of services provided. As the continuum of care evolves, the focus will shift to integrated models where all care providers, enrollees, payers, and community share the risk, cost, as well as the gain on outcomes mutually agreed upon as a part of their involvement. With the shift to health status versus illness, new measurement designed to show preventive outcomes along with morbidity and mortality data will be needed. Outcome evaluation should include how we are servicing people in healthy ways rather than only documenting what went wrong and what has not worked. Another key point to consider while designing a measurement model is that the health care system is built around illness care focusing on about 10 to 15 percent of the population, leaving 85 to 90 percent of the population without effective outcome measures. As new models are created and healthy status is the desired outcome, consideration will be required for those in the 85 to 90 percent [group].

• Supporting New Behaviors in the Desired Culture

As transformational processes are institutionalized, it will be necessary to reward and reinforce the new behaviors of the desired culture. Focusing on rewards for small successes as well as larger breakthroughs allows everyone in the organization to feel needed and that he or she is a "winner." The strategic elements of many innovative projects carried out by SHNP project teams are reward, recognition, and celebration. For example, Tallahassee Memorial Regional Medical Center planned a graduation ceremony that showcased and celebrated the accomplishments of the center's "start-up" teams (operational and clinical improvement teams). District of Columbia General, University of Cleveland Hospitals, Harbor-UCLA Medical Center, MeritCare Hospital, and St. Luke's Regional Medical Center all included leaders from their human resource departments early in the change process to plan and implement reward, recognition, and compensation systems appropriate to emerging new roles and work. They planned hospitalwide celebrations to mark significant stages along the change process journey. During these events, everyone is recognized, which emphasizes the importance of the people who perform the day-to-day work.

Harbor-UCLA Medical Center's restructuring initiative is based on the philosophy that an internal sense of community with stakeholders using leadership practices is necessary to achieve shared organizational goals and personal accountability. Leaders at the center believe that "everyone is a member of the campus community; everyone is a leader and a stakeholder, including patients and their families." In order to institutionalize its philosophy, the medical center designed a We Care Week, which is a celebration coordinated by its Community Initiative Strategic Direction Council, an interdisciplinary group that is part of the center's community design model. Events and objectives include:

- *Come Meet Our Community:* To introduce members of the community to each other, including internal members (administrators, managers, physicians, nurses, support staff, patients and their families) and external members (vendors and business people). This event presents an opportunity for hospital personnel and community members to learn about each others' contribution to improving the community's health status.
- *Celebrating Our Harbor Community Past, Present, and Future:* To recognize and celebrate the institution's history and diversity.
- *Customer Service Day:* To provide education and training on how to talk and relate to customers, creating partnerships between customers and campus employees.
- *Taste of Harbor:* To celebrate the Harbor community through the tradition of food, celebrating the diversity of their culture. Some call this "meet[ing] the community through a cookbook."
- *Employee Recognition Day:* To provide an opportunity to have fun at work through dressing in nontraditional ways; to formally recognize groups and individuals as outstanding members of the community.
- *Harbor Fair and Picnic:* To provide the opportunity for community members to meet and know each other in an informal, fun atmosphere.[9]

Called a Community of Patient Care Leaders, the model is based on the following components:

1. *Community initiative:* A organizational spirit that emphasizes the sense of community in all aspects of organizational life
2. *Leadership culture of continuous improvement:* An organizational culture characterized by leadership initiatives among all stakeholders at all levels of the organization
3. *User-friendly environment that empowers stakeholders:* An environment that empowers individuals and supports the mission of the organization through effective and integrated systems
4. *Systems to facilitate transitions:* An expectation that systems are identified to support transitions (adaptation to change) for all stakeholders.[10]

• Conclusion

Transformational leaders expect tension and conflict as part of the change process, and they stress reward, recognition and celebration as essential components. As organizations undergo change, management structures move from traditional, dependent hierarchies to those of collaborative, interdependent models and circular designs. These participative structures support involvement of all stakeholders, thereby aligning them with the organization values and purpose.

References

1. Peck, M. S. *A World Waiting to Be Born: Civility Rediscovered.* New York City: Bantam Books, 1993.

2. Gilmore, T. N. Dilemmas of institutionalizing transformations. SHNP education program, Orlando, FL, Sept. 1993.

3. Gilmore, T. N., and Krantz, J. Innovations in the public sector: dilemmas in the use of ad hoc process. *Journal of Policy Analysis and Management* 10(3):455–68, 1991.

4. Stetler, C. B., and Charns, M. P. *Collaboration in Health Care: Hartford Hospital's Experience in Changing Management and Practice.* Chicago: American Hospital Publishing, 1995.

5. Ackoff, R. L. *Creating the Corporate Future.* New York City: John Wiley and Sons, 1981.

6. National Program Office. *Strengthening Hospital Nursing: A Program to Improve Patient Care National Meeting Brochure and Meeting Resource Notebook.* St. Petersburg, FL: Robert Wood Johnson Foundation and Pew Charitable Trusts, 1994.

7. Improving patient care at Penn State-Hershey Medical Center: unlimited Horizons. *Strengthening* 1(4):3, 6, Winter 1995.

8. Patton, M. Q. *Practical Evaluation.* Newbury Park, CA: Sage Publications, 1982.

9. National Program Office.

10. National Program Office.

Part Four

Addressing the Challenges of Change

• Introduction to Part 4

Taking personal responsibility is important in society where blame belongs to the next person and where people consider themselves smart when they take all they can get. Leadership is best set by example. . . . Examples of personal responsibility are what could make the difference in charting new directions. Responsibility is a sign of transformation.

The Soul of Politics, Jim Wallis

The challenges of organizational transformation, especially in health care, are formidable. What is the vision of the new health care system, and what values do patients and payers expect? What new and improved relationships will help realize opportunities to add value? Which structures support those relationships? Can the values and structures of old models and practices carry us into the future? How can we align ourselves and the organization with its destiny? Is the new system based on altering the future by remembering the past and transforming the present?[1,2] How can the personal dignity, individual contribution, and aspirations of everyone be respected and nurtured as we care for the soul of persons and the organization? How can people take personal responsibility and teams learn collective accountability during times of turbulence and uncertainty?

One of the greatest enemies of creating a resilient work force is doubt — self-doubt and doubt in others.[3] Recognizing that an organization's most valuable resource is its people, transformational leaders work to overcome people's doubts and encourage their self-mastery. They look for the potential in people and try to help them satisfy their aspirations through trust and respect and by believing in them and having confidence in their outcomes. They encourage new and improved interpersonal relationships, and they mentor others to become leaders. Transformational leadership is an art that requires practice in valuing the talents and knowledge of others and supporting behaviors that promote success.[4-6]

Part 4 consists of two chapters that look at the human and system factors that challenge transformational leaders. Chapter 8, Addressing the Human Factors in Change, describes behaviors that promote success and those that prevent it. People resist change in different ways and sometimes exhibit sabotaging behaviors that may be messages from leaders as well as other employees or stakeholders. The chapter concludes with a discussion of how the roles of different hospital leaders — physician, board members, and executive nurses — are being affected by the change process. Chapter 9, Addressing the Systems Factors in Change, addresses systems factors that require attention in order for an organization to respond to its market area quickly and consistently. These factors include human resources, information systems, and financial systems. Transformational leaders show how they are reaching to new constituents, including educational institutions, policymakers, legislators, and payers as they restructure their systems to create and deepen interdependence and interorganizational relationships.

References

1. Wallis, J. *The Soul of Politics.* Maryknoll, NY: The New Press and Orbis Books, 1994.

2. Hammer, M., and Champy, J. *Reengineering the Corporation: A Manifesto for Business Revolution.* New York City: Harper Collins Publishers, 1993.

3. Stewart, T. A. How to lead a revolution. *Fortune,* Nov. 28, 1994, pp. 48–61.

4. Stewart.

5. Covey, S. R. *Principle-Centered Leadership.* New York City: Simon & Schuster, 1992.

6. Senge, P. M. *The Fifth Discipline: The Art and Practice of the Learning Organization.* New York City: Doubleday, 1990.

Chapter 8

Addressing the Human Factors in Change

Cornerstones of civil behavior: (1) the capacity, on both the individual and the corporate level, to distinguish between necessary, legitimate suffering and that which is unnecessary or excessively convoluted; and (2) the willingness to bear that suffering which is a proper portion in both our individual and corporate lives.

A World Waiting to Be Born: Civility Rediscovered, M. Scott Peck

The process of group or team formation has been described by many, including Scholtes[1] and Peck.[2] The stages of this process can be traced through the evolution of organizations undergoing change and include shifts from pseudocommunity to chaos to a cohesive unit effectively working together. In the early stages of the change process, politeness prevails. Over time, however, profound individual differences emerge that produce chaos as people either adjust to the differences or attempt to obliterate them. Ultimately, people no longer retreat from the differences but, rather, absorb and work with them in an attempt to connect with each other through dialogue to achieve common meaning and purpose.[3-5]

This chapter looks at the impact of change on the organization from the human perspective. It identifies strategies that may be used to overcome resistance to change among the hospital's general population and examines how the roles of key executive leaders must change in order for organizational transformation to be successful.

• The Human Response to Change

The human response to the notion of change is complex. Some people readily embrace it; others resist with every fiber of their being. Resistance is a normal response to change and an expected behavior during the developmental stages of organizations or groups undergoing transformation.

Levels of Resistance to Change

In an effort to understand resistance to change, Martin Charns, member of the SHNP National Advisory Committee, has noted that there are three circles of acceptance in a typical organization. Each of these circles comprises about a third of the organization's population. He found that there are:

1. *People who are champions of transformation:* These are people so deeply invested in the process and outcome of change that they cannot imagine another way of doing things. They are forever optimistic and see opportunity in everything; they see problems as challenges to be overcome while reaching new potentials. They are cheerleaders with enormous energy, eager to move forward.
2. *People who take a wait-and-see approach:* These are people who think they might invest in the change but are unwilling to commit right away. However, once these people have an "Ah ha" experience (discussed in chapter 5), they often are stronger supporters than those in the first circle. Although they may have agreed with the desired outcome from the outset, they had to accept the process for themselves and understand their personal accountability for the outcome.
3. *People who refuse to invest in the change:* No matter how hard people in the other circles try to persuade them, these individuals will not endorse or invest in the change.

Considering the overall goal of the change process, transformational leaders must decide whether to keep the people in the last group within the organization or to offer them career counseling that would enable them to pursue other occupational options. The decision as to whether to keep them or encourage them to leave should be made after assessing whether their resistance could be a contribution to the change process and desired outcome. Sometimes resistance can be viewed as an opportunity for growth by members of the other two circles because people who resist change often raise probing questions or point out undesirable consequences of change that need to be considered. Acknowledging their value to the team effort may soften their attitude and help them understand that they have a contribution to make. However, individuals who continue to show a resistive attitude and behavior eventually will sabotage team efforts. In such cases, the better option will be to counsel these individuals to leave the organization.

Annette McBeth, vice-president, Immanuel-St. Joseph's Hospital, likens the process to that of riding on a moving train:

> Teams have a collective energy and creativity generated by the diverse ideas and imagination of the members. Their energy fosters enthusiasm throughout an organization as they move forward in the direction of

their shared vision. To illustrate this point, as the train moves along the track, energy begins to build. People will either choose not to participate or to champion the innovation and climb on board. The conductor, at some point, must say to those people who choose not to participate — either climb aboard or look for an alternative work environment. If people choose alternatives, they must be allowed to do so with dignity.

However, it also is important not to misinterpret the reasons for resistance. Marianne Araujo, senior manager, Ernst and Young Consultants, cautions that "resistance to change is different depending on the level within the organization that the resistance occurs and the position of the person resisting. It may not be that the intent is to be resistive but, rather, that two parties do not agree on the same goals. It may not be resistance to change; it may be the failure to believe in the change." In some cases, resistive behavior reflects a lack of proper understanding of the desired outcome.

Strategies to Overcome Resistance

Transformational leaders recognize that individuals accept and understand the need to change differently, and thus plan and implement strategies to enable everyone to work through dissimilar feelings and perceptions. They encourage use of a variety of tools to deal with resistive behavior, including conflict resolution, communication processes, assertiveness training, grieving processes, and continuous improvement techniques. The common factor among all these tools is interactive conversation and dialogue which lead to deeper acceptance of the why of resistance by all parties. Stories, parables, metaphors, and games also may be used to make a strong or difficult point. Such strategies enable individuals to become enmeshed in the essence of the meaning of change through imagination and creativity, providing them with a way to work out feelings before dealing with the real situation. Interactive communication skills such as listening and dialogue should be used to develop trust and establish integrity to create a functional relationship between persons leading the change and those resisting it. Some leaders advocate assigning a support person to an individual experiencing difficultly. Edward Foley, regional vice-president, Hospital Council of Southern California, explains this approach when dealing with current senior-level management:

What do you do when members of the senior management team do not have an "Ah ha" experience? Some just don't, or won't. Nonetheless, these can become full participants in the change; it is just not their style or personality makeup to have you share in how they go about understanding and accepting major shifts in accepted paradigms for your hospital or corporate culture. These people should not be made to feel they are less a part of the program because they have not shared a "conversion experience" with others. Treating them evenly with colleagues who may be more exuberant about paradigm shifts will be a key to bringing them into new behaviors and assuring their effective participation.

Thomas Mroczkowski, vice-president/COO, Hackley Hospital, describes the same approach when bringing a new senior-level manager into the organization:

> We first invest significant time up front during the interview process. A potential new member of Hackley Hospital's leadership team is interviewed both singly and in groups by potential peers and associates. The interview is designed to assess the applicant's ability to embrace our organizational culture, as well as their technical ability to do the job. Once hired, the new member is assigned to a mentor who is responsible for showing them the ropes and insuring that the individual receives basic leadership development orientation, as well as a basic leadership skill assessment; that includes taking a leadership effectiveness analysis and brain dominance test.

• Behaviors That Promote Success and Those That Sabotage It

Often people's responses to the change process are influenced and sometimes determined by their leaders' behavior. Leaders who believe in the change send messages that promote support for the change process; those who do not support the change often send messages that can sabotage the change effort. Sabotage is one of the most effective ways to deter successful change. It may be planned or unplanned, conscious or unconscious, with or without intent. Following are aggregate lists of behaviors or role messages that can lead to success and sabotage collected from various transformational leaders.

Role Messages from Executive Leaders

Transformational leaders report that when executive leaders (for example, CEOs, nurse executives, and trustees) demonstrate the following behaviors, they promote support among employees for the change process. An executive leader will send messages that can lead to success if he or she:

- Believes in the project; lets go of traditional thinking
- Mentors the personnel responsible for the process and implementation

- Supports unit staff involvement, ensuring attendance through resource allocation
- Supports risk taking, willingness to experiment with new ideas; tolerates failure; and encourages creativity and imagination
- Integrates the project with other institutionwide strategic initiatives
- Keeps project visible to the board of trustees
- Keeps informed of national and local issues
- Involves all disciplines and departments, focusing on the organization as a whole
- Provides adequate resources, space, people, time
- Is a cheerleader; takes an active, visible role, including attending meetings
- Assists other management staff in understanding the importance of the scope of change, reinforcing that change is okay
- Delegates decision making to the lowest level possible
- Is prepared to focus discussion and to be the person to receive the blame for institutional shortcomings; is prepared to be alone

However, executive leaders also sometimes demonstrate behaviors that send negative messages to employees. Ultimately, these messages will deter success. An executive leader sends messages that will sabotage the change effort if he or she:

- Talks only one discipline (for example, nursing)
- Is indifferent toward those potentially affected by the outcome
- Treats new ideas as things that cannot be done; holds on to the past
- Ignores existing organizational values
- Talks too much, dominates discussions, and makes decisions for the group
- Gives inconsistent messages and withholds supportive resources
- Neglects to redirect an individual's functions outside the project when that individual is given added responsibility for the project
- Isolates other disciplines and does not encourage their involvement
- Inserts red tape or does not troubleshoot for team
- Is too protective of his or her personal vision
- Has a predetermined idea of the answer
- Fails to get out of the way, to involve the right people, to take risks, and to accept failures

Role Messages from Physicians

Another group whose behaviors send positive or negative messages to employees is that of physicians. A physician sends positive messages that will support change if he or she:

- Identifies key medical staff and other medical team members, such as residents

- Promotes the project at medical staff functions and encourages involvement
- Emphasizes the impact for the improvement of patient care
- Develops milestones with planning team, documents success, and shares information
- Encourages physicians to learn the work and roles of other caregivers
- Promotes collaborative practice and problem solving
- Accepts ideas from others, listening to understand their message

The physician who demonstrate the following behaviors sends negative messages. He or she:

- Takes a passive or trivializing attitude
- Maintains a traditional "physician in charge" role
- Uses support of the project as negotiation leverage
- Insists upon autonomy
- Fails to communicate to medical colleagues
- Is closed to change

Role Messages from SHNP Project Directors

The last group to report was that of SHNP project directors. Their behaviors also send messages that can either promote or sabotage project success. The project director whose behaviors send positive messages is one who:

- Gives up personal agendas, or makes them equal to the agendas of others on the team
- Establishes a climate of invitation to participate, versus mandated participation
- Actively seeks change, encourages those who are reticent
- Defines expectations and responsibilities for persons involved
- Maintains a timetable and communicates it to everyone
- Strives for neutral identity when discussing issues
- Provides structure to keep the process on track
- Focuses on idealized vision as well as details

The SHNP project director who exhibits the following behaviors sends negative messages. He or she:

- Does not share credit for accomplishments or acknowledge input from others
- Stays too busy with day-to-day activities
- Submits to individual desires instead of the group's desires
- Does not reframe content for different participants or loses the focus of the objective

- Acts as an elitist
- Fails to include individuals who may be affected by the outcome
- Is too active in the process; imposes personal ideas; is afraid of the risk of failure
- Falls into old ways of thinking about the organization
- Loses patience with noncooperative or resistive people
- Does not share the vision; is secretive
- Proceeds primarily with ideas from known opinion setters

• Impact on Organizational Transformation by a Change in Leadership

Senior-level leadership changes are a common occurrence today. Some organizations strategically prepare for recruitment of a new leader by involving managers and unit-level staff along with physicians and trustees in the recruitment process. Identifying characteristics and values compatible with the mission and management practices of the organization allows these stakeholders to feel pride in the selection of a new leader who has the potential to share their beliefs. At Hartford Hospital and Harbor-UCLA Medical Center, the departing leaders provided input into the recruitment process. The Harbor-UCLA outgoing CEO also participated in the new CEO's orientation, thus ensuring a comfortable transition in leadership and an understanding of the organization's transformational processes. Organizations recruiting a leader in the more traditional manner by using the board of trustees as the primary selection mechanism experience difficulty in transitioning to new leadership styles. One organization in the SHNP experienced three senior leadership teams in a two-year period. The original team, which valued interactive and interdependent processes, horizontal integration of interventions, and developmental programs for staff at all levels of the organization, initiated the change process. But selection of the new CEO was made by the board with limited input from the remaining senior team members. The new CEO brought in her own team of senior leaders who were traditional and authoritarian in management style, and there was no strategic plan for blending their style with the participative management style of the original team. Many difficulties ensued, including loss of trust by physicians, nurses, and other professionals for administrative practices, and confusion and frustration among staff. Morale dropped and staff reverted from patient-focused approaches to department-focused behaviors. When it became apparent that the second leadership team would not be effective, its members were dismissed and a new team was recruited. Key staff members were involved in that interview process along with board members, and the third team was compatible with the desired future for the organization.

Araujo explains that the principles behind the decision to effect organizational change must remain constant during the process of managing a change in leadership:

These principles include identifying and articulating the mission and values, constant infrastructure, a measurement process, and an overall desired outcome for the organization. For effective change, these elements should remain constant unless there is collaborative agreement and supporting information that indicates a need to alter them. For example, a decision to merge institutions or a management buyout may create a need to change one of the fundamental principles. Elements that can change are the means and resources to carry out the change, the developmental processes, and the systems to be improved.

Even organizations experiencing significant leadership change can continue revolutionary ideas if the founding principles are constant. However, they are encouraged to plan for and select successive leadership. A lack of a strategic effort may result in resistance and even sabotage to an innovative process. This becomes particularly disruptive when unit-level staff, middle management, physicians, and trustees have endorsed the innovative initiatives and infrastructure. Traditionally when there is change in top-level leadership, particularly the CEO position, the leader will bring her or his ideas and possibly team members who have a similar style. The new leaders may impose their ideas and style on the organization. Organizations that are experiencing transition from an authoritarian to a participative approach may become confused and dysfunctional if new leadership is not compatible. Early in the transition, people are vulnerable and skeptical. If new leadership moves in during that stage of the transition and they have not embraced the change principles, the organization may take many steps backward and experience a difficult time rebuilding trust and introducing collaborative approaches. If new leaders desire trust and acceptance of their ideas and style, it is important for them to acknowledge and appreciate the organizational history. Organizational history does not begin with their joining the organization. A leader who is sensitive to the people and history of the organization will prepare everyone that the management style will shift according to her or his style. People will have an opportunity to choose to work within the organization as it is newly defined or pursue other options. Sabotage occurs when direction is not clear, people no longer feel valued, or the destination is whimsical versus clearly defined. Participative change can be stopped as a result of a leadership change.

• Impact of the Change Process on Senior Leaders

Physician, trustee, and nurse executive roles all are influenced by the change process. These positions need to be involved early on in the process, including the initial developmental activities. The following subsections describe how each of these roles is affected.

The Physician Role in the Change Process

As mentioned previously in this book, because physicians tend to feel they have greater insight into the clinical work of the hospital, they are the most likely of the senior leaders to resist taking the time necessary to become part of the team process until they have been assured of the benefit of the change for them and their patients. However, many physicians indicated that once they could see the effect of change for patients and improved efficiencies for themselves, they readily and enthusiastically endorsed and championed the change. Therefore, to encourage physician participation in and support for the change, the institution may have to employ certain strategies. For example, physician department chairs from University Hospital/ Pennsylvania State University, The Milton S. Hershey Medical Center, in Hershey, Pennsylvania, initiated interactive planning and management techniques and systems principles in department operations and teaching functions with residents and medical students.

Richard Lindsay, head of the Division of Geriatric Medicine, School of Medicine, University of Virginia, suggests the factors and strategies that apparently encourage physicians to participate in the change process:

> It usually is related to the personality of the individual — a person who has been chosen by his or her peers to lead quality improvement efforts. Often it is a senior, well-respected physician with a long record of hospital leadership. In some institutions, it is a physician identified by nurses as someone who is seriously interested in designing better clinical care programs. In other instances, it is a physician whose practice would clearly benefit by the new methods and attention. The stature of the physician leader makes the difference. . . . If a busy practitioner begins to tell his or her colleagues about the benefits of new patient care programs, this is positive and encourages interest and involvement by other physicians.
>
> It is key to ensure that physicians are involved from the initiation of a clinical improvement project. They need to feel that their input has been sought and represented from the project's inception. Survival of the institution often is a key motivating factor in physician involvement with successful revision of patient care processes. When physicians and others take part together in patient care committee work, patient care improvement works especially well. Managed care also definitely helps to pull physicians and hospitals together. This process is stimulated by market share and regional alliances.
>
> Clearly the adage of keeping one's eye on the ball seems to be the answer. If patient care is the ball, leadership can bring together the team

of transportation, nursing, laboratory, maintenance, admitting, X ray, housekeeping, pharmacy, record room, dietary, and safety to improve the process of patient care. This interdisciplinary process, accompanied by individual empowerment, must replace the old barrier of departmental structure that has impeded revision and improvement of the care of patients. Patient care processes in the hospital are inexorably linked with the patient care processes outside the hospital and are an essential ingredient for system success. Some institutions fail to capitalize on the opportunity to carry out improving patient care outside the hospital walls by integrating the practicing physicians offices as well as community service agencies. If, in the hospital setting, departments can replace the myopic viewpoint of solely meeting the needs of their departments, with one of collaboration including physicians meeting the needs of the patients and their families, an institution is on its way to successful change. It is in this setting that the unit-level staff understanding of some of the problems involved in hospital care of patients can finally surface and the true meaning of empowerment is realized. For example, a patient need-driven belief is made operational when admitting office hours are changed to meet the needs of working patients rather than the needs of admitting office staff, a change suggested by employees from the admitting office at one successful site.

Interactive processes, systems thinking, interdisciplinary involvement, and quality improvement should be integrated processes in order to realize institutionwide improvement for patient care outcomes. Nurses, physicians, and other staff require systematic development and education in these processes before they can be institutionalized.

The Trustee Role in the Change Process

The role of the board of trustees in protecting and promoting the mission and values of the organization in partnership with management, medical staff, and the community is essential.[6] A well-defined mission, specific strategies to carry out the mission, and systematic training of board members, including new trustee orientation to institutionwide innovations and goals, are necessary elements for success.[7-9] Overall, the board must ensure hospital management's ability to focus on the bigger picture, including the needs of the community, through involvement in strategic organizational projects.

As a former board member for Health Resources Northwest, in Seattle, Washington, and a consultant to hospital and health care system boards, Winnie Hageman, principal, The Umbdenstock-Hageman Partnership, describes the necessity of board involvement in the change process:

> Board members who are oriented to the hospital project and its goals are enthusiastic and feel ownership for the outcomes. They share information

with their colleagues and are an ambassador for the innovations of the hospital in the community. As new members join a board, full orientation to the mission and strategy of the change process is essential. Empowering those closest to the work is critical to the success of the project, but leadership at the top cannot be abdicated if real change is to occur. The board may not be intimately involved in the project, but their commitment to its success can help sustain the process, even with changes in executive leadership. They are committed to a vision of being the best tertiary care medical center in their area of the country with particular sensitivity to the health care needs of their region. Also, the importance of community commitment cannot be overemphasized.

Peggy Hughes, secretary, board of directors, Tallahassee Memorial Regional Medical Center (TMRMC), adds to discussion of the necessity of trustee involvement in the change process by describing the interaction between the board and staff at TMRMC:

My role as a board member is to be a conduit from the steering committee (governing body for the interactive management model) to the board of directors. I also represent the board at unit-level graduations (Startup) and poster presentations. [Startup teams are interdisciplinary unit and department teams that have formed a unit and department board, identified their problem list, and implemented an intervention to resolve the problem. Once a team has completed its work, it celebrates with graduation and hospitalwide poster presentations.] During these presentations, I am able to hear directly from unit staff how the interactive process helped them accomplish patient care and system improvements. The sense of ownership for the redesign of the work on their units is impressive. I believe my interest and participation affirms their efforts as I share with other trustees their enthusiasm for patient care improvement outcomes.

As interactive training is institutionalized and unit-level staff initiate the process, I am aware that dialogue rather than discussion has been occurring at the unit level with everyone having a sense of shared meaning. There is ownership of the corporate vision and an understanding that what is done on the unit level builds bridges toward achieving the vision. Dialogue is couched in terms of vision and the language of the interactive process. That language and the resulting understanding of the process is permeating the corporate body.

The board is revisiting the mission statement at least yearly. The mission statement is our corporate vision, and the board has the responsibility to keep the vision large enough so everyone can feel ownership, including the community. The mission statement provides a new framework within which the board can evaluate how the organizational efforts achieve the shared vision. My liaison role allows the board to be informed by one of their peers, and enhances their understanding of how staff are becoming more creative and less reactive in thinking.

One of the most exciting outgrowths is the empowerment of individuals who have participated in the learning process. Employees articulate that living the vision is possible not only in the corporate culture but also in personal life. Having a personal vision helps create a personal reality that an individual desires for [him- or herself]. Individuals, as well as corporations, can mentally rehearse the future; when we focus on the results we want, our minds can make that future happen. We can be empowered, individually and collectively, to be the architects for building a healthier community.

Chris Beebe, board of trustees, Northeast Health Consortium, first provides a list of ingredients for a successful relationship between the board and leaders of the organization and then describes the value of being part of a consortium:

- *Trust:* To enable collaboration and productivity in pursuing common goals for the health care system
- *Education:* To facilitate appropriate and sound decisions
- *Commitment:* To stand up for what is right for the shared mission
- *Vision and mission:* To stick to the larger picture, allowing management to handle the details and give them the freedom to accomplish the stated mission
- *Risk taking:* To chart unexplored waters and move ahead
- *Clarity:* To have dialogue; listen to and learn from each other

My role as a board member changed when I realized the value of the consortium. Through working together, we could create an integrated community health care system, as opposed to a scattered bunch of health care delivery systems — facilities that were tied together legally but not operating in a unified and efficient way. Insight occurred as we assessed our separateness and understood how inefficient it was to have four different boards. The challenge was to facilitate the same kind of thinking with others. Many continued to see separate boards and facilities. They wanted the security of being together, but they did not want to give up autonomy. We started with open, honest conversation focusing on what we wanted — an integrated health care system in mid-coastal Maine. Using the interactive process and an outside consultant, the four boards and senior facility leaders committed time and energy to identify our shared vision and strategic action steps. Building trust over time is critical to the transformation of any board. Transforming means change; change occurs only if people trust one another enough to have dialogue. Once a board is clear on what is right and each individual can live with the agreement of what is right, the next step is to have a group that is willing to take the risk and say "Let's do it." I do not think it is reasonable to expect to have 100 percent approval on a decision; 80 to 90 percent is plausible.

The outcomes that I hope we achieve as a consortium are to be responsive to patients and their families as needs change and services are integrated between facilities. Community health care, if it is to be integrated, must embrace all disciplines and all services. Board members and executive leadership working together will facilitate transformation to embrace not just medical care but health care in the truest sense. The most successful health care systems will be those that see the broad picture including the contribution that can be made to the health status of the community. They will be the ones that implement cost efficiencies through shared resources by carrying out a unified mission.

Trustees are challenged to balance professional life with the needs of the organizations they support. They also must manage conflict between personal needs and the needs of the community as a whole. These can be addressed through dialogue and involvement in the organizational operational process. Additionally, board members have accountability for translating economic and social objectives into cost and quality (value) strategies that enable the organization to grow and thrive. Thus, they must be knowledgeable and informed and have the time to develop trust with multiple stakeholders, including physicians and other professionals. In the transformation, they will be involved in numerous interorganizational relationships involving integrated delivery or service networks. These relationships may have multiple objectives including defining capital needs, achieving political and social legitimacy, procuring greater market share, and providing better service to the community.[10,11] Transformational leaders recognize that trustees represent the interest of the community health status, and view the board as ambassadors not only for the organization but the community as a whole.

The Nurse Executive Role in the Change Process

Of all the leadership roles affected by the change process, perhaps the nurse executive role is the one most affected. Nurse executives pursuing transformational values and characteristics must balance the economic forces of the organization with high standards of professional practice while advocating for patients and their families. Experts in clinical care processes, they must be able to combine their talents and competencies with other professionals to develop collaborative and cocreator relationships that support a patient-centered continuum across care settings. Although managed care and capitated reimbursement systems may alter how nurse executives function, they will not alter their responsibility to sustain excellence in patient care practices.

Dominick Flarey, administrator/COO, Youngstown Osteopathic Hospital, describes the role of the nurse executive in the transformation of health care:

> The introduction of the prospective payment system was the real turning point in the transformation of the role of the nurse executive, along with other leadership roles. This era requires health care systems to focus more intently on how care is being delivered. It ushered in the cost and quality imperative. Nurse executives are most expert in the delivery of care and became pivotal in the quest for an ongoing transformation. Of all health care executives, the nurse executive understands the business of health care down to the cellular level. Because of this, nurse executives play a major role as internal consultant to the executive team and board of trustees.
>
> The nurse executive brings to the table many skills and much expertise. Perhaps the greatest of these is the inherent understanding of interactive planning and systems thinking. In clinical training and practice, nurse executives are ingrained with the interactive planning process. They are taught to envision outcomes for patients and plan backwards to the realization of such outcomes. Nurse executives are experts in planning and it is this expertise that is pivotal in the ongoing transformation of health care. Nurse executives have a profound understanding of systems. Their clinical training and background is heavily concentrated in the understanding of the person as a system, made up of multiple subsystems. This includes the effects on the entire system when there is malfunction in one or more subsystems. Nurse executives understand that subsystems must work together for there to be optimal health. They are able to transfer this clinical knowledge and experience to the function of a health care system. This, coupled with their intense understanding of the business of care delivery, places them in a powerful and influential position within the organization.
>
> The majority of changes that have occurred in the delivery of health care services over the past decade have been initiated and driven under the leadership of the nurse executive. One example is case management, which evolved from pressure on nursing leadership to deliver high-quality, cost-effective services under the mandate of the prospective payment system by reducing patient length of stay. Other examples include the integration of care that has occurred from the acute, inpatient setting to home health services and the innovative redesigns in care delivery systems that are occurring across the country. No other role has

undergone such rapid transformation over the past decade as that of the nurse executive. They are emerging as primary transformational leaders in this era of health care, and I believe that it will be the nurse executive who will play the primary role in moving our health care systems forward.

Sharon Lee, vice-president, patient care services, St. Luke's Regional Medical Center, explains how her position has been affected by the change:

My position evolved from a traditional line executive, senior vice-president for nursing, to a staff position, vice-president for patient care services. Now, rather than representing only nursing, I have responsibilities to represent all patient care providers within the employee structure for St. Luke's Regional Medical Center. This role change provides me an opportunity to promote an interdisciplinary approach to the delivery of patient care rather than a discipline-specific approach. While I have no operational authority for the business centers of the organization, I have influence on the clinical processes of care delivery based on standards of care and identified clinical outcomes. The power to create change and affect decisions comes from my ability to influence based on knowledge and expertise, not from formal organizational authority. In the new organizational structure, the humanistic aspect of building relationships is essential to partnerships with physicians and community providers of health services.

• Conclusion

The human response to change varies from individual to individual. At either end of the spectrum, people accept it wholeheartedly or resist it wholeheartedly. Realizing the range of acceptance (or resistance), transformational leaders initiate strategies early in the change process to prevent or minimize potential interference with a successful transformation. However, whether employees exhibiting resistive behaviors are kept in the organization or encouraged to find other career options, transformational leaders treat them with dignity and respect.

The change process can likewise be seriously affected by changes in senior-level leadership. When a senior leader such as a CEO leaves the organization, whether or not the new leader's selection and orientation involves key stakeholders at all organizational levels can make a major difference between a smooth or turbulent transition in management style. Additionally, the organization must consider the impact of the change process on its senior leaders. Physicians and trustees need to be informed and involved throughout the change process, especially in the earliest phases, because their willingness and ability to form collaborative relationships can affect the success of the change. Their roles, along with that of the nurse executive, seem to be the ones most affected by the movement from hospital-focused services to capitated care and community-focused services.

References

1. Scholtes, P. R. *The Team Handbook.* Madison, WI: Joiner Associates, Inc., 1992.

2. Peck, M. S. *A World Waiting to Be Born: Civility Rediscovered.* New York City: Bantam Books, 1993.

3. Isaacs, W. N. *Taking Flight: Dialogue, Collective Thinking, and Organizational Learning. Dia•Logos.* Cambridge, MA: Organizational Learning Center at Massachusetts Institute of Technology, 1994, pp. 24–39.

4. Peck.

5. Schein, E. H. *On Dialogue: Culture and Organizational Learning. Dia•Logos.* Cambridge, MA: Institute for Generative Learning and Collaborative Social Change, Inc., 1994, pp. 40–51.

6. Umbdenstock, R. J., and Hageman, W. M. *Critical Readings for Hospital Trustees.* Chicago: American Hospital Publishing, 1991.

7. Drucker, P. F. *Managing for the Future: The 1990s and Beyond.* New York City: Truman Tally Books/Dutton, 1992.

8. Drucker, P. F. *The Five Most Important Questions You Will Ever Ask about Your Nonprofit Organization.* San Francisco: Jossey-Bass, 1993.

9. Umbdenstock and Hageman.

10. Umbdenstock and Hageman.

11. Drucker, 1993.

Chapter 9

Addressing the Systems Factors in Change

This is not the beginning of the end. It is the start of the next cycle; a whole new era in providing community-based health care with a formula that emphasizes capitation, clinical protocols, ambulatory care, noninvasive surgery, and substantial reliance on nonhospital settings such as subacute and home care. Health care can learn a lesson from these companies seeking to reinvent themselves: (1) create vision and leadership; (2) put customer needs first, especially the need for security; and (3) move quickly to implement new strategies. Every day spent in waiting to confirm trends before taking a new direction is going to be very costly.

> Russell C. Colile, Jr., Looking forward.
> *HOSPITAL Strategy Report* 7(1), Nov. 1994

Institutions seeking operational efficiency in response to market demand are creating integrated health care networks, or organized delivery systems, by redefining services internally and forming alliances externally. These institutions are finding that horizontal integration produces cost containment strategies, such as group purchasing and consolidating system functions, that are achieving efficiency by increasing the size and scale of operations. They also are finding that vertical integration results in the delivery of seamless, better coordinated care through establishment of clinical protocols, practice guidelines, and case management with programs that emphasize wellness and prevention.[1-3] Integrated health care systems profit enormously from centralizing information services, unifying managed care contracting, and merging financial structures by pooling revenue, assets, and debt.

This chapter looks at systemic factors that are essential to successful systems integration. It also identifies barriers to systems integration and offers premises for future decision making suggested by a number of contributing transformational leaders.

• Integrated System Development

In *Creating Organized Delivery Systems: The Barriers and Facilitators,* Shortell and colleagues discuss the key strategic characteristics of integrated health care systems, which include breadth, depth, and geographic concentration.[4] *Breadth* refers to the number of different services and functions provided along the continuum of care, including the extent to which insurance components are offered. *Depth* refers to the number of different operating units within a system that provide a given function or service. *Geographic concentration* refers to the extent to which operating units of the system are located in proximity to each other.

These characteristics are important because they help determine the size and configuration of a delivery system. Stakeholders of successful networks consider how much of the continuum to provide in terms of breadth and assess how to activate the continuum in terms of depth and geographic concentration based on population needs and the presence of local competing systems. Some degree of breadth across different levels of care is required to promote vertical integration, and some degree of depth is required to promote horizontal integration. For example, an established integrated health system offering a wide array of services across the continuum of care (breadth) is more easily able to partner with additional providers of needed specialty services (depth), such as a well organized home health agency seeking a wider market area.

Other aspects of an integrated system include:

- *A resilient work force* that can adapt to changing roles and positions within the organization
- *New covenants* between people within the organization and between the organization and entities in the community
- *Accurate information systems* and real-time databases that can be used to manage more effectively
- *Social accountability* assumed by transformational leaders involved with integrated delivery financial systems

These are discussed in the following subsections.

A Resilient Work Force

Transformational leaders recognize that the human element is an essential part of the change process as organizations move into a new system. They are aware that people within the organization worry about how the change is going to affect their job security, seniority, and need to master new procedures and techniques. One way to foster resilience among the people of the organization and to build their trust is to open channels of communication early in the process.[5,6]

Resilience is the ability to (1) work in different roles and locations within the system and (2) accept the challenges and interferences of system formation as opportunities to achieve the system's destiny, which is to promote a healthier community.[7,8] Every organization has the resources and means within it to create a resilient work force. Its leaders can promote resilience by providing supportive environments that enhance readiness for change and provide clear and continuous information.

Resilience also can be achieved in part through developmental processes that clarify how individual contributions are valued by the organization and how stronger relationships within and outside the institution will help achieve desired outcomes. Wayne Frieders, vice-president, human resources, St. Luke's Regional Medical Center, and Linda Fleury, human resource analyst, MeritCare Health System, stress that:

> . . . the power of developing strong trusting relationships and having a commitment to an organizational vision and purpose that is larger than any one individual or department is critical to establishing and maintaining a resilient work force. Employees need to understand that if difficulties arise such as cost reductions, their managers will respect their dignity even when tough decisions have to be made. When the culture is one of trust and respect, employees are apt to take responsibility and accountability for systems improvement potentials; they realize their role in cost efficiencies and do what they can to contribute, including retraining for new roles and sometimes leaving the organization.

Development of a resilient work force also includes a dynamic role for educational institutions at all levels. For example, Tallahassee Memorial Regional Medical Center, in Tallahassee, Florida, and Health BOND, a partnership between hospitals and higher education in south central Minnesota, both used interactive management processes and system thinking principles as they collaborated with a variety of educational institutions including elementary schools, high schools, colleges, and universities in determining present and future work force needs.

Geraldine Felton, professor/dean, College of Nursing, explains what is being done at the University of Iowa to make this collaboration effective:

> The national and state health system reform agendas are infinitely complex. These agendas and related issues have begun to impact a variety of areas of the university because of extensive involvement in the provision of health services, the need to educate health professionals, and engagement in basic, applied, and clinical research in the health sector. At the University of Iowa, we are challenged to devise creative solutions to the complex issues of providing service, doing research, and providing health care workers with the skills, values, and attitudes necessary to work

in a different type of health care world. We simultaneously strive to foster new partnerships among the professions and with the community, redefine our mission to serve community needs, bring creativity and innovation to the educational process and work environment, and produce educational programs that are demanded by students and future employers. We are reaching out to new constituents and welcoming them into the process of recreating the mission and direction of the institution. By doing so, we create new political and economic alliances that will assist us to do what we need to do to contribute to better distribution of health manpower. That needs to start with three things:

- A mechanism to facilitate analysis, information sharing, and coordination of agendas among the many individuals in various organizational units of the university with those who are involved in health system activities at the state and federal level
- A forum whereby university positions and/or specific legislative proposals can be formulated, refined, and adopted related to important aspects of national and state health system reform
- A process to assist in university efforts to transmit a common message to policymakers and our constituents regarding curriculum, use of resources, and issues of the health system reform agenda as they relate to the missions of the University of Iowa and the general societal good

Interdisciplinary strategies are increasingly the only valid pathways to address the complexity of the problems. In reaching out to new constituents, and creating alliances, coalitions, and partnerships, the hope is that such strategies will lead to more effective sharing of resources and more creative responses to problems. The investment is expected to produce new approaches to teaching, learning, and clinical practice. New relationships are built by ensuring that education, formal and informal, is centered on value-centered lifelong learning; and by communicating the need to explore and critique the relationship between professional values and the changing health care system. If the professions are to be preserved from becoming just associations for health care workers, then their work must begin and end on the fundamental values that define and shape their calling. Education, perhaps more than any other institution affecting the professions, is in a position to form these values initially, to reinforce them throughout professional life, and to reinterpret them with the demands of health care change. We are beginning to agree on the overreaching standards of commitment and belief and what these standards mean for our academic health center. They form an "ultimate concerns model" for ethical thinking to keep in mind when making decisions. These are the value statements on which we propose to maintain our balance in an uncertain world:

- Society has an obligation to assure that individuals receive necessary health care.
- Limited societal resources for health care must be allocated so as to provide maximum quality of services at a socially acceptable cost.
- Within their capabilities, individuals are ultimately responsible for their own health and their health-related behaviors.
- Reasonable consumer freedom and opportunity for choice among health care options and courses of treatment must be preserved.
- Health professionals must be educated and function within a context of shared values.
- The Academic Health Center must be responsive to the health needs of the public and the well-being of our communities.
- The health care system, and Academic Health Centers in particular, must encourage and stimulate innovations that enhance access, improve service quality, and promote the efficient utilization of resources.
- The fundamental role of the Academic Health Center must be to generate, disseminate, and apply the knowledge that improves human health and the quality of life.

New Covenants

As organizations create integrated networks, transformational leaders recognize that new covenants are needed between employers and employees, boards of trustees and managers, health care institution and health care institution, and health care institutions and communities. These new covenants must include shared maintenance of and responsibility for enhancing the quality of work life and the soul of each employee. For example, working with trustees, transformational leaders need to provide the tools, environment, and opportunity for assessing and developing the skills of everyone involved in cocreation of the system. They are responsible for operationalizing a common framework that everyone understands, with common indicators across the system to measure outcomes. This framework includes a common financial and clinical language that is customer focused and service driven and that ensures a uniform system of financial reporting from the top level to the unit level. As a clinical framework, it ensures that all care providers work in a meaningful manner to achieve success for themselves, the patient, and the system. Development and implementation of this framework is facilitated through use of a variety of work and role redesign tools and techniques.[9] These techniques will be selected using interactive management, systems thinking, and learning organization principles. Additionally, they will be based on the mission of the network or system and designed to achieve value-driven outcomes.

Additionally, as integrated delivery systems evolve, there no longer will be simple staff roles primarily learned on-the-job. Rather, human resource professionals will be challenged to prepare employees to develop problem-solver and opportunity-identifier skills using management and staff development techniques.[10] Opportunity-identifier skills are used in the interactive management process to identify the gap between current reality and the desired outcome (chapter 4). Principles that guide these human resource functions include:

- Ensuring that everyone in the system understands its mission and values
- Monitoring current system skills and talents to recruit for future competency gaps
- Training and developing system stakeholders in skills and talents that customers demand, ensuring that quality is maintained in the learning process
- Facilitating the transfer of knowledge (learning organization principles) throughout the system by designing and implementing programs that enhance a flexible work force able to be reassigned to positions throughout the system

Often visionary thinking or revisioning about future system requirements can help define current system opportunities and enhance the process of designing current interventions or inventions as described in chapter 4 through the interactive management and planning process. For example, the Staffing Network of Vermont, an interhospital staff-sharing system that coordinates access to nurses and other health care professionals and technical employees, is looking to the future. It is developing a vertically integrated model to share staff among different types of providers in smaller rural communities. This model demonstrates a covenant between the community hospital and a local home health agency to improve the health status of the community. Visionary plans also are under way to enhance information systems and develop a comprehensive database that can be accessed quickly and easily by hospitals and other facilities statewide.

Accurate Information Systems

Without the integration achieved by information systems (IS) and the real-time databases they provide, integrated networks will not be able to manage effectively. Information systems are needed to track populations and enrollees and to focus on their health status indicators.

Bill Sonterre, vice-president, acute care systems, describes the vital role of information systems in keeping connected the various elements of the integration network at Abbott-Northwestern Hospital. He also discusses some of the challenges facing information systems:

Abbott-Northwestern is creating an environment with intelligent, multi-functional workstations that have full access to all clinical support systems including laboratory, pharmacy, radiology, registration, medical records, point of care (patient bedside computerization system), electronic mail, and other data pertinent for clinical support. An "electronic highway" between service and support areas is the network infrastructure (local area and wide area) that connects all areas of the hospital together, as well as connecting the hospital to all other care-giving facilities across an integrated service network. Abbott-Northwestern is now a member of Allina Health System, a health delivery network of more than 17,000 employees, 7,000 contracted providers, 17 hospitals, 45 clinics, 580,000 members of Medica managed care products and nearly 300,000 members of Select Care's preferred provider organization. In order for a health system network to achieve integrated services, information systems has to be the glue that links and meshes clinical and financial management systems into a seamless, user-friendly support environment. Senior management has to define priorities for IS and in doing so recognize that IS can be helpful in the following ways:

- Quantifying and tracking benefits realized by the use of information technology
- Supporting training efforts, both delivery of training, such as multimedia portable computers located on care provider units, as well as providing systems for tracking and maintaining training records
- Working with innovation and quality improvement project teams to organize systems requirements, conduct systems evaluations, and coordinate and collaborate in vender selection and contract negotiations
- Ensuring agreed-upon criteria and performance expectations with users for pilot tests and documentation of those performance criteria prior to final acceptance of new systems or technology
- Supporting projects such as point of care systems; shared registration between hospitals, clinics, and physician offices; coordinated patient scheduling across the health care campus; and nursing LAN, a decentralized communication system for nurse managers used for staffing functions and other management strategies

A challenge facing information systems is the shifting of scarce resources from traditional financial business applications to the direct support of patient care delivery. Critical to this shift is the performance evaluation of information services. In the past, such evaluations were unstructured giving little direction for future strategic choices. Now, with the advent of network delivery systems, applications are selected to build on and enhance the IS profile and the user's functionality. As expensive clinical information and management technology is considered, a formula should be developed and agreed on by senior management, along with care providers and other users such as payers, for providing the appropriate IS personnel to support the investment. Without full support the potential of IS will not be realized, nor will the users of the systems be satisfied.

As hospitals become a part of integrated delivery networks, it is cost-effective and efficient to share learnings and experiences across member organizations. For example, the nurse manager LAN from Abbott-Northwestern is being developed for United Hospital in St. Paul, Minnesota. A major challenge for large enterprises, such as Allina, is to strike a balance between the enterprisewide strategic initiatives and site-specific innovation and redesign activities. The challenge is to tie these together so they do in fact support each other. Employing professionals on the IS staff that come from the clinical disciplines, such as nursing and pharmacy, is of great value when it comes to understanding the care delivery process for specific patient populations and arriving at improvements to the process for individual sites as well as the entire system. Since joining Allina, collaboration is strengthened across organizations in order to actualize site-specific and total system improvements. If the information system is to transition effectively and efficiently to support clinical systems, health care organizations also must design salary structures and benefits for IS personnel that are competitive with other industries such as banking, retail, and insurance.

The strength and commitment of the IS group often can be identified in the shared vision of the group. The shared vision during this transitional process for the Abbott-Northwestern information service reads "our mission is to deliver to every employee and caregiver the information they need to be able to do their job as efficiently and effectively as possible."

Sonterre adds to his look at the role that information systems currently play in integrated networks by assessing the role they will play in the future:

Mergers, acquisitions, partnerships, and the rate of technology change have an enormous demand for IS to adapt rapidly and deploy new systems, integrate systems, and convert systems. Strategic priorities include efficient and cost-effective support of numerous hospitals, clinic sites, and physician offices toward common core systems including patient registration, order-entry management, laboratory, pharmacy, radiology, medical records, and financial systems. An important goal for ISNs is to create a computerized patient record. At this time, there is no magic answer to building the ideal computerized patient record. It will require a major effort by many people from a variety of clinical disciplines and support to assemble the components. Standardization and integration of patient/client clinical data across clinics, offices, hospitals, and eventually the home is absolutely essential for efficient and efficacious patient care. As health care reform unfolds, it will be critical to reduce customer hassles and improve customer access. This will require customer-friendly, seamless access across the ISN. Key components such as customer master index, enterprisewide patient scheduling, patient or client identification, and smart cards responsive to the customer's ability to move from facility to facility across the enterprise all will be a part of the intercommunication highway.

Efficiencies and quality will be enhanced by the standardization and collection of enterprisewide basic financial and clinical management information. The data are essential for analysis, decision making, and determining IS performance and strategic priorities. Enterprises will require systems and technology allowing physicians user-friendly linkages and easy access to clinical information across the enterprise. These linkages will augment their services, improve quality patient outcomes, and enhance their ability to compete in the managed care market. Collaboration and partnerships with physicians will be required to achieve mutual benefits for the care provider, ISN, and the patient.

Enterprisewide networks and applications infrastructures will include local area networks, wide area networks, and worldwide Internet access. Regional, state, and national health care electronic highways will evolve to a state of common, everyday usage. Applications such as common electronic mail systems are rapidly becoming a part of each care provider and support person's work life. Close partnerships with key information or communication system vendors will be required to meet the needs of the diverse components of a large enterprise. Flexible designs that are easily tailored and customized will be a priority as vendors are considered for these partnerships. The success of the system may be in proportion to the investment in planning and evaluation of the IS profiles, the support to the system, and the ease of customer service. It is expected that the capital budget supporting IS will increase 5 to 7 percent or higher over the next few years. Although change will be required in a timely, responsive, possibly rapid manner, senior management should plan strategically how rapidly new technology can be deployed. As the Allina Health System relationships mature and stabilize, leaders have learned that there is a limit in how much "change an organization can deal with at one time."

Confidentiality of patient or client data will grow as a major issue as ISNs form and integrate services across care settings. A paradox will exist since there will be a demand by both the consumer and care provider to know all the care being delivered and to have readily available any significant clinical information that would aid and improve the care delivered while maintaining confidentiality in the process. Resolution to this issue will not be easy and it will require the collaborative efforts of health policy personnel, insurance carriers, and providers along with transformational leaders who have a sense of social accountability.

Social Accountability

Transformational leaders involved with integrated delivery financial systems will assume social accountability along with systems performance accountability. According to Mark Burzynski, president/CEO, Yellowstone Community Health Plan, this means that as care reaches into the community the hospital serves, new "integrated financial systems will be needed which address outcomes of this continuum." Chief financial officers (CFOs) will become mentors, teaching teams how to manage resources so as to deliver higher-quality services more efficiently to patients and families. (See chapter 1.) They will become attentive to the health status of patients and the community, as well as to the requirements of customers such as vendors, payers, and educators. He asserts that the effectiveness of managed care programs will depend not solely on contracts, payment plans, utilization review, and so on, but also on the relationships that providers build with the communities they serve.

Thus, community values and service gaps (perceived and potential) will be a part of the strategic performance plan. Managed care competition will continue to require that systems have reliable cost-of-service data to remain viable with likely future erosion of profits. The CFO will have a significant role to play in networks determining how organizational performance can be maintained while providing a value outcome for the community as perceived by both consumer and payer.

John Romas, J.A.R. and Associates, and Annette McBeth, vice-president, Immanuel-St. Joseph's Hospital, elaborate on the need for integrated financial systems as the continuum of care is extended beyond the walls of the hospital:

> Tracking the health of an individual rather than inpatient bed use, admission data, or type of service will be an essential part of the transition to a new financial systems. Comparing the cost of service provided versus the cost of prevention will be another essential element. The systems will focus on cost factors for maintaining a healthy status for the individual and the community, rather than on illness. This focus will be influenced by the relationships which care providers have with enrollees, relationships purchasers have with each other, and the relationships that the community and the payers have together. Attention will be given to sharing the risk, cost, and gain between providers, purchasers, and payers of health services. The transition will be an empowered approach, with people taking responsibility and accountability to improve or maintain

cost efficiencies and value. This shift to empowerment should positively impact family health, community health, and beyond. Providers and payers working together in a coordinated effort have the potential to address social issues effectively. Through their collective efforts they will decrease the cost relating to resolving those issues and enhance the health status of the community.

Bob Siver, vice-president of managed care, All Children's Hospital, adds to the discussion by describing the reasons for the public demand for managed care and the physician's role in the process:

Someone must decide issues of access, appropriateness, quality, and cost of health care. These individuals must understand principles of economics and financial systems and temper them with social accountability. Managed care organizations are consolidating power rapidly in the market, and lobbying statements of politicians are taken seriously by those with the authority to change reimbursement distribution. Along with financial systems knowledge and skills, leaders need to facilitate changes of attitude, particularly with physicians regarding managed care. The window of time for attitude change is small. The American public has demanded managed care for three reasons:

- Resources are not unlimited.
- All care is not appropriate.
- All care is not of high quality.

Computer networking capabilities give instant dissemination of laboratory and radiographic testing results and make possible an electronic medical record and nationwide data banks for outcomes and treatment protocols. Where is the physician in this process? Few physicians understand or utilize the existing rudimentary computer capability already existing in their hospitals and offices. This is to abdicate information systems development to others who do not always have the needs of the patient and physician clearly in mind. Physicians need to work closely with executive leadership to develop computer skills and management knowledge to contribute to integrated models of care currently emerging to meet the need of community wellness rather than the illness-centered models of the past. Physician executives are needed for appropriate clinical input into hard decisions that need to be made today. The bottom line in all of this for everybody, especially physicians, is performance—the delivery of value for the patient and the payer. Value is a combination of competitive price and high quality. The test over time will be performance and value.

• Barriers to Successful Systems Integration and Formation

Shortell and colleagues also have discussed the major barriers to integration and system formation, offering suggestions for overcoming each.[11] All the system's stakeholders, including physicians and trustees, are influenced by these barriers, which are commonly seen in all merger and alliance activity and are cited by numerous contributors to this book. The primary barriers to successful systems integration or alliance formation include:

- Understanding that the new core business of health care is (1) primary care supported by preventive care and (2) maintenance care organized to deliver improved value to patients and payers
- Overcoming thinking in terms of the hospital–campus model and shifting to a community-based systems focus
- Helping the "cash cow" facility to understand that (1) the new health care environment is broader and requires new alliances with possible former competitors and (2) debt may need to be shared among system members
- Accepting that changing roles, relationships, and responsibilities of management, care providers, and trustees in the new system may make many positions and functions ambiguous, including the need for physicians to fill management roles
- Managing care effectively to (1) negotiate capitated contracts that generate prepaid revenue for the system and (2) utilize advanced practitioners appropriately in primary care settings
- Creating relationships that meet requirements of the customer as core strategies
- Developing system unity while maintaining individual uniqueness of member facilities that serve diverse populations
- Utilizing effectively the talents, knowledge, and skills of a culturally diverse work force while paying attention to the soul of the individual and the work force's connectiveness to the organization and community
- Fostering new relationships that provide opportunities which liberate people to be who they are and to fulfill their destiny

Many multi-institutional health care systems, including Mercy Health Services, University Hospitals of Cleveland, Northeast Health, Providence Portland Medical Center, and the PROMINA Health System, are overcoming barriers and implementing innovative relationships with their communities by forming coordinated longitudinal continuums of care services among hospitals and other care settings in their market areas. The following subsections describe how each of these systems is achieving this.

Mercy Health Services

Mercy Health Services (MHS), a multi-institutional consortium located in Michigan, Illinois, and Iowa, has developed 15 community health care systems (CHCSs) that focus on community-based integrated delivery of care. Each CHCS has a unique model and approach for integrating services across the continuum from acute care to home care, long-term care, and preventive care, including specific services for the aging. The goal is to improve community health status by increasing the efficiency and efficacy of patient care using existing resources. Common themes are:

- Collaborative practice models featuring case management across the continuum of care
- Staffing models to facilitate multidisciplinary care teams
- Integration of innovations through clinical information systems
- Improved quality measurement
- Shared education across facilities

Additional hallmarks are involvement of community members in defining health care needs and specifications of the community-based model; strengthening of relationships with academic counterparts in colleges and universities to create relevant curricula and practice designs; and system-wide development of futuristic information systems to establish real-time clinical, financial, and management databases. MHS has initiated and implemented a number of strategies to prepare for future challenges and opportunities. The MHS Professional Nursing Practice Plan clarifies nursing practice throughout the CHCS, and the Physician Blue Ribbon Panel provides vision and structure for physician involvement across the entire continuum of care.[12]

University Hospitals of Cleveland

In Ohio, University Hospitals of Cleveland, a 947-bed academic health center, has created affiliates in four counties surrounding Cleveland, including Lorain Hospital in Lorain County; Lakewood and Marymount Hospitals and University MEDNET, a multispecialty group practice with three ambulatory sites, in Cuyahoga County; Geauga Hospital in Geauga County; and University MEDNET in Lake County. Affiliate hospitals range in size from 169 to 350 beds and serve rural and urban areas. The network includes:

- Collaborative care processes with integrated clinical pathways for specific patient groups
- Work and role redesign for nurse case managers and support staff

- Skills-based training for leadership to support learning organization principles
- A central structure and function to support innovation and clinical excellence throughout all institutions[13]

University Hospitals tests models considered for collaboration before sharing them with affiliates, and adapts them to meet local environmental forces and patient populations. The system and MEDNET analyze outcomes for improving health care for their communities while creating cost efficiencies through integrated care processes. The network system is challenged with strategic cost reduction activities requiring human resource redistribution from inpatient to ambulatory settings; more efficient use of technology; and diversification to meet the demands of a turbulent market in the greater Ohio area, which is undergoing multiple mergers and management changes. According to Nikki Polis, project director, University Hospitals and Network Hospitals, "Early involvement in network collaborative efforts of physicians and other stakeholders, along with new financial and clinical information systems, strategic planning, and market research strategies, has contributed greatly to University Hospitals' current success."

Northeast Health

Northeast Health, a consortium of institutions in Maine focusing on the continuum of care between acute care, long-term care, and home care members, is developing an integrated clinical delivery system based on case management and clinical pathway strategies using centralized information services (IS). One motivation for developing the system was the increasingly elderly and economically high-risk population the consortium serves as it prepares to manage the care of patients for whom high costs are anticipated. Consortium members have established innovative partnerships with payers to provide well-coordinated care for patients and their families in the most cost-effective environment. For example, Blue Cross and Blue Shield, which formerly reimbursed only for emergency or inpatient care for children with asthma, has agreed to reimburse for ambulatory care. This change in policy has reduced cost and enhanced satisfaction because parents learn to manage the care of the child at home. Patient outcomes also have improved because parents have learned how to recognize conditions that may trigger asthma episodes and how to manage episodes earlier.

Providence Portland Medical Center

Providence Portland Medical Center is sharing leadership and educational resources throughout the Sisters of Providence Health System in the northwest region of Oregon. The vision statement supporting this redesign effort is: "To use patient needs, expectations, and the achievement of quality patient outcomes for the redesign and improvement of health care delivery." Its quality improvement and redesign restructuring focuses on relationships with patients, care providers, managers, the community, and payers; and builds on the values of quality, service, flexibility, efficiency, empowerment, and involvement and learning throughout the system. The framework guiding day-to-day implementation stresses teamwork, multilevel involvement, accountability, continual improvement, data-driven decisions, and new processes and systems to achieve predetermined desired outcomes. The Sisters of Providence Health System continues to explore ways to coordinate and manage care and services for populations throughout the region. A longitudinal trajectory to achieve vertical integration guides this work, and includes the processes of access and entry, wellness, prevention care, acute intervention, chronic care, transitional care, and long-term care.[14]

PROMINA Health System

In Georgia, in October 1994, the Gwinnett Health System, the Northwest Georgia Health System, and Piedmont Medical Center created the PROMINA Health System, an alliance of more than 2,500 physicians and 10 "not-for-profit, for-people" hospitals in the greater Atlanta metropolitan region, including a full-service psychiatric hospital, senior congregate living facilities, comprehensive home health services, health and fitness centers, and multiple urgent care, multispecialty, and freestanding primary care centers. The three objectives of an initial "bottoms-up" off-site, weekend strategic planning conference involving 80 selected stakeholders, including 27 physicians, were:

- To agree on a common vision
- To build the PROMINA team by developing personal relationships among team members and becoming more knowledgeable of the organizations that comprise PROMINA
- To develop consensus on long-term strategic directions and short-term strategic initiatives

Breakout work sessions were held in three areas:

- Managed care (analyzing local, metro, and state markets)
- Vertical and horizontal integration opportunities
- Operational efficiencies

The resulting vision statement is "to measure and continuously improve the health status of our communities by developing and operating an integrated health system, offering a full continuum of high-quality, cost-effective services, with a commitment to wellness, patient-focused care and education." Implementation is proceeding at a rapid pace with centralization and expansion of information services as a top strategic priority.

• Premises for the Future

As health care industry leaders prepare for the future, contributors report that, independent of national- and/or state-legislated policy changes, they are transforming institutions to create responsive, effective, efficient, high-quality, and value-centered health care systems for their communities and market areas. Following are some of the premises that will guide their activities:

- Capitation will be the predominant form of paying providers of care.
- Competitive providers will form strategic alliances including collaborative partnerships and cooperative networks.
- Integration of health care institutions into systems or networks with physicians and payers will increase.
- New incentives for maintenance care, wellness, preventive care, education of all stakeholders, and related efforts to reduce utilization will be widespread.
- Competitive pricing of network services will precipitate unprecedented cost reductions because of economies of scale of large systems.
- Primary care will reign supreme as the most influential force in health care decision making.
- Practitioners prepared at an advanced level, such as nurse practitioners and physician assistants, will assume greater roles and responsibilities in areas of patient care formerly reserved for physicians.
- Work force resiliency will free management to grow and develop the business.
- Self-care information and tools will have primary importance.
- Reward and reinforcement for lifestyle improvement will be a part of the health care dynamics.
- Community-based continuum of care networks will be the principal means of overall cost reduction and quality enhancement, increasing value to patient and payer.
- Destiny and soul of the work force and system will be recognized.
- Relationships to identify and realize new opportunities will be made and strengthened.

• Conclusion

In addition to addressing the human factors in change, institutions desiring to undergo transformation also must consider the systems factors in change.

Systems factors are those involved in the formation of integrated health care delivery networks, or organized delivery systems. Such networks or systems will require development of a resilient work force; establishment of new covenants among managers and employees, hospitals and hospitals, and so on; implementation of accurate information systems and real-time databases; and assumption of social responsibility by leaders involved with integrated delivery financial systems. To achieve their vision and overcome inherent barriers to system integration, institutions will have to apply proven strategies and take into consideration premises identified by transformational leaders and stakeholders across the country as guidelines for future development.

References

1. Drucker, P. F. *Managing for The Future: The 1990s and Beyond.* New York City: Truman Tally Books/Dutton, 1992.

2. Shortell, S. M., Morrison, E. M., and Friedman, B. *Strategic Choices for America's Hospitals: Managing Change in Turbulent Times.* San Francisco: Jossey-Bass, 1992.

3. Spath, P. L. *Clinical Paths: Tools for Outcomes Management.* Chicago: American Hospital Publishing, 1994.

4. Shortell, S., Gillies, R. B., Anderson, D. A., Mitchell, J. D., and Morgan, K. L. Creating organized delivery systems: the barriers and facilitators. *Hospital and Health Services Administration* 38(4):447–66. Winter 1993.

5. Connor, R. D. Bouncing back: resilience as the essential component that transforms the reality of organizational change into a manageable process. *SKY* 23(9):30–34, Sept. 1994.

6. Waterman, R. H., Waterman, J. A., and Collard, B. Toward a career-resilient workforce. *Harvard Business Review* 72(4):87–95, July–Aug. 1994.

7. Bolman, L. G., and Deal, T. E. Merger meltdown. *Healthcare Forum Journal* 37(6):30–36, Nov.–Dec. 1994.

8. Connor.

9. Hanson, R., and Sayer, B. *Work and Role Redesign: Tools and Techniques for the Health Care Setting.* Chicago: American Hospital Publishing, 1995.

10. Schmeling, W. *Becoming a Health Care Learning Organization: Building the Capacity for Continuous Change* [working title]. Chicago: American Hospital Publishing, 1995.

11. Shortell, Gillies, Anderson, Mitchell, and Morgan.

12. National Program Office. *Strengthening Hospital Nursing: A Program to Improve Patient Care National Meeting Brochure and Meeting Resource Notebook.* St. Petersburg, FL: Robert Wood Johnson Foundation and Pew Charitable Trusts, Fall 1994.

13. National Program Office.

14. National Program Office.

Part Five

Looking at Those Who Have Experienced Change

• Introduction to Part 5

> The corporations, for their part, have engaged in a willful battle against the grain of existence. . . . They have spent enormous amounts of energy putting in place systems that attempt to hold back the shifting oceanic qualities of existence.
>
> *The Heart Aroused: Poetry and the Preservation of the Soul in Corporate America,* David Whyte

In the past, the complexities of leadership often could be lessened simply by incorporating instructions in the organization's operating manual or promoting the teachings of the latest workshop on management. However, the problems of leadership in health care reform cannot be solved so easily. In order to design a desired future that values the health status of the community, organizational leaders will need to draw on their own imagination, insight, and creativity; and may need to use nontraditional sources such as poetry to stimulate and engage institutional imagination and creativity.[1] From the boardroom to the unit level, the use of imagination encourages organizational accountability to the community the organization serves,[2] and transformational leaders not only accept that accountability but expect it in their work force.[3] Leaders ask for new and improved relationships and attentiveness to the soul of the organization by demonstrating respect for, and trust and belief in, the organization's most important resource — its people. By seeking opportunities supported by their vision, transformational leaders want to deliver improved value and to fulfill a destiny more meaningful than that of making financial profit. Building a shared vision is the starting point for organizations or health care systems hoping to achieve this. Vision begins in "open space." Once it is shared, it has the capacity to focus and galvanize the spirit of the people and organization in remarkable ways;[4] and leaders are able to liberate their work force to be self-directed as they focus on growth and development of the organizational business — the organizational destiny.

Part 5 presents the experiences of six organizations in the throes of transformation to improve health services in their communities. Each has leaders who embrace interactive planning and management, systems thinking, value framework concepts, and learning organization principles. Each has developed a shared vision at different times using different methods; and each has institutionalized its vision as the guiding force for defining opportunities for change and selecting appropriate interventions (inventions) to implement change. All are encouraging new and improved intra- and interorganizational relationships among their people.

Chapter 10, University Hospital of Utah, and chapter 11, Providence Portland Medical Center, discuss planning processes, supporting infrastructures, and the desired value of improvements for patients and their families, care providers, and the organization. In an appendix, this chapter includes comments from patients who were involved in focus groups during the planning process. Chapter 12, Health BOND, describes this consortium's partnership between service and education in south central Minnesota. The partnership is based on a shared governance model and leadership principles fostered through a Leaders Empower Staff Education and Training Program provided for members of the partnership. In chapter 13, District of Columbia General Hospital, and chapter 14, Vanderbilt University Medical Center, key leaders provide insights gained through their involvement in innovative processes for patient care delivery. They also comment on leadership style and role functions with the involvement of key stakeholders, including physicians. Chapter 15, Northeast Health Consortium, discusses the importance of communication and collaboration as leaders in mid-coast Maine design an integrated care delivery system between an acute care facility, long-term care, home care, and the community.

References

1. Whyte, D. *The Heart Aroused: Poetry and the Preservation of the Soul in Corporate America.* New York City: Doubleday, 1994.

2. Morgan, G. *Imaginization: The Art of Creative Management.* Newbury Park, CA: Sage Publications, 1993.

3. Whyte.

4. Owen, H. *Leadership Is.* Potomac, MA: Abbott Publishing, 1990.

Chapter 10

University Hospital of Utah

Located in Salt Lake City, University Hospital/University of Utah Health Sciences Center (UH), a 388-bed academic medical center, developed a new strategic planning process with the objective of redesigning patient services to (1) provide high-quality, cost-effective care across the continuum of service and (2) improve the supply and utilization of professional resources. This chapter describes UH's new approach to strategic planning and the three innovative programs that evolved. A significant component of the project team's planning process is the use of patient focus groups, which is explained in the appendix to this chapter.

• UH Approach to Strategic Planning

Historically, University Hospital's board of trustees set direction for the hospital's strategic planning process. Each department initiated processes focusing on new program development with a two-year perspective. For example, the nursing practice department (NPD) initiated its process through a council that organizes staff representatives according to job classification — from general staff through nurse executives. The council identified and prioritized annual goals through a serie of council retreats. Although this approach allowed for flexibility and input from a variety of sources within the NPD, no mechanism was in place to bring NPD recommendations together with those of other departments in order to design programs that would benefit the overall organization and, ultimately, the community.

In 1988, the NPD, with the support of executive leadership, launched a new and different kind of strategic planning process. The new process initially focused on redefining the role of the professional nurse. Influenced

Chapter 10 was prepared by University Hospital's Program to Improve Patient Care staff Susan Beck, RN, PhD; Evelyn G. Hartigan, RN, EdD; Cheryl Kinnear, RN, BSN; and Jackie A. Smith, PhD by the nursing shortage of the 1980s and patient care demands resulting from increased intensity of patient illnesses and technological advances, the NPD defined the role of the clinical nurse to more appropriately utilize his or her professional knowledge in the care of patients. Extending the perspective to the year 2000, the NPD placed emphasis on defining roles for both the professional and technical work force.

Recognizing That Relationships Are Key to Change

Desiring to strengthen nursing to improve patient care and knowing that all professional caregiver roles are changing, the NPD designed UH's Program to Improve Patient Care: An Interdisciplinary Collaborative Process for Change. The NPD realized that strengthening one profession would affect all other institutional health care professionals. Thus, recognizing that professional relationships would be the key element of change and acting in accordance with SHNP objectives and the interactive planning concepts of Russell Ackoff, the NPD decided to move from the boundaries of nursing service to the broader dimensions of patient care services involving caregivers from all disciplines and departments, including patients and their families. The willingness of individuals throughout the hospital to embrace this new way of planning set the stage for institutionwide acceptance. As Susan Beck, nurse researcher and project director, explains: "The potential to work together, with staff crossing departmental lines, created new excitement and energy."

A shared organizational vision to improve patient care became the hallmark for the future, moving the NPD away from improving separate departments and disciplines to strengthening the entire organizational purpose. The new challenge became one of trying to initiate a program without departmental or professional boundaries in the creation of an integrated care delivery system across the entire continuum of inpatient and outpatient services. The designated project team, which included executive leaders and caregivers, began to "de-institutionalize" many outdated practices to achieve new features and values based on everyone working together. The new, integrated organizational structure and the interactive nature of the process were fundamental to the project's ultimate success.

Building on the Existing Chain of Command While Empowering Multidisciplinary Task Forces

As the approach to strategic planning became institutionwide, the project team used the concept of stakeholder management to identify who should be involved in the process. *Stakeholder management* identifies, involves, and manages stakeholders — those individuals, groups, or organizations that have a stake in or are affected by what the organization wants — in other words, its desired outcome. Looking at UH's mission and role in the community, the team identified both internal and external stakeholders. (See figure 10-1.) *Internal stakeholders* were defined as those individuals who operate primarily within the walls of the medical center, and *external stakeholders* were defined as those who operate outside the medical center's walls and are affected by what it does.

Stakeholders actively participated through an integrated structure involving both new and existing hospital groups. (See figure 10-2.) The intent was to build on the existing chain of command while empowering multidisciplinary task forces of managers and staff to generate options for patient care improvements. New groups included a project advisory committee (PAC), a strategic planning team (SPT), a steering committee, and task force groups. The PAC included external stakeholders, UH leaders, and project staff. Its role is to set direction for the project based on the health care needs perceived by the stakeholders of the medical center and University of Utah campus, state-level organizations, local and state government, and the Salt Lake City community and surrounding area. This group also advised the

Figure 10-1. Map of Internal and External Stakeholders

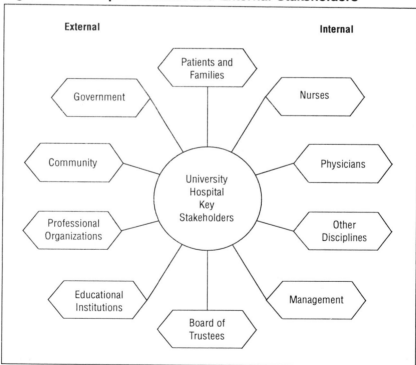

Source: University Hospital's Program to Improve Patient Care, University of Utah, Salt Lake City.

Figure 10-2. New and Existing Strategic Planning Groups

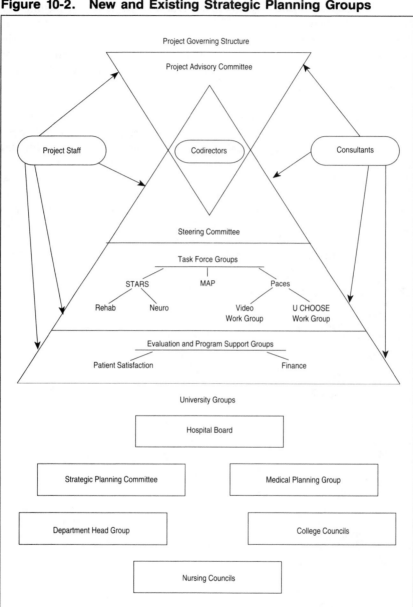

Source: University Hospital's Program to Improve Patient Care, University of Utah, Salt Lake City.

project team on changes in national health care policy that could influence institutionwide strategic planning. The SPT mixed internal stakeholders from all levels of the organization representing operational and clinical functions. The steering committee was composed of a representative group of leaders from SPT, including senior management, medical staff members, department directors, and project staff. (Figure 10-3 shows the makeup of these committees.) SPT members, along with key members of the PAC, were given training in interactive processes. Hospital executive staff committed the necessary resource support such as secretarial time, clinical staff and manager time, office operations, and data collection tools and processes.

As planning evolved, the level of stakeholder involvement was extended to five task force groups, which further refined and developed specific ideas and action plans. Because members of the hospital chain of command (existing groups) were also members of the new PAC and SPT groups, they served as liaison between the existing and new integrated structures. The new structure became the organizational support for patient care innovations directed by the UH project team. It exists as a parallel system to the existing chain of command.

Figure 10-3. PAC, SPT, and Steering Committee Membership

Project Advisory Committee	Strategic Planning Team
State legislator	UH board member*
Deans of College of Nursing, School of Medicine, and College of Pharmacy	CEO/codirector*
Faculty in health economics	Chief nurse executive/codirector*
Professor/endowed chair in health policy	Associate administrator, professional services
Representative, Church of Jesus Christ of Latter Day Saints	Medical staff representative*
Presidents, Utah Nurses Association and Utah Medical Association	Director, planning and marketing*
Executive director, Utah Hospital Association	Director, nursing research*
Representative, health department	Director of nursing, home care
President of UH medical board	Director, ambulatory care services
Project director, quality improvement consortium	Clinical director of nursing
Representative, SHNP National Advisory Committee	Representative, head nurse, staff nurse, and clinical manager
UH CFO	Representative, managed care
Project director and codirectors	UH controller
	Director, respiratory therapy
	Director, pharmacy
	Faculty, College of Nursing
	Representative, quality assurance
	Project director
	* Steering committee members

• Framework for Participative Interactive Planning

Guided by interactive planning (IP), the SPT created a desired future. The stakeholder structure—PAC and SPT—provided the framework for participative planning. Stakeholders learned and applied the idealized design process to identify ideas, attributes, and characteristics of the desired patient care delivery system—a system that valued patient-centeredness, the continuum of care across services, appropriate use of a professional work force, and satisfaction for patients, their families, and caregivers (including nurses, physicians, and other stakeholders). "Knowing what we wanted," reports Beck, "we planned 'backwards' to realize that delivery system." IP was implemented in six stages:

1. *Understanding the perspectives of key internal and external stakeholders:* A variety of methods were used to collect data on the perspectives of key stakeholder groups or, in IP terms, "formulating the mess." Five focus groups met with former UH patients who identified two needs: (1) improve continuity of care through better coordination and consistency of caregivers and (2) improve communication by providing information about expectations and care before, during, and after hospitalization. Interviews and meetings with nurses, physicians, and other hospital personnel also indicated two issues: (1) A significant portion of professional time was spent in work that could be performed by nonprofessionals or support workers, and (2) many professionals and departments were providing services to the same patients, even though each area was organized to deliver care in a different way. Thus, an inordinate amount of time was being spent by care providers communicating and attempting to coordinate care, and patients and their families were feeling confused as a result of not knowing what to expect when they needed inpatient services.

2. *Generating the idealized design or desired patient care delivery system:* The SPT used a process consultant to facilitate IP learning, develop relationships among multiple disciplines, and formulate strategies on how to work together. Team members attended a two-day retreat to accomplish stages two and three. Three work groups were formed to generate the idealized design (stage two) for delivering patient services, each of which was assigned one of the center's three primary mission components: patient care, education, and research. The groups were asked to complete an exercise based on this premise: "UH has been destroyed. You are part of a team asked to design a new hospital using your assigned mission component as a basis for planning." Nominal group technique was used to ensure that SPT stakeholders could equally and fairly contribute to the idealized process. Each group identified qualities, attributes, characteristics, and behaviors of this new hospital, and the ideas of all groups were displayed. Using the mission components facilitated

identification of innovations specific to a teaching institution. It also helped people understand their common purpose and begin removing programmatic boundaries that discouraged their working together.

3. *Challenging assumptions, practices, and traditions:* In this stage, stakeholders were asked to challenge assumptions, practices, and traditions underlying the ideas, attributes, and characteristics identified for the idealized design. Using lateral thinking techniques as described by E. deBono,[1] they surfaced their challenges. The groups moved to a new level of interaction and creative thinking. For example, one person said to another: "You're assuming that our service begins on the day of admission, what if we could begin before that?" This resulted in people imagining beyond current constraints, boundaries, and rules of hospital structure; and created an environment in which everyone had the opportunity to challenge current practices and traditions and to consider the potential of what could be. New and exciting ideas emerged, and relationships among care providers began to form.

4. *Prioritizing the ideas, characteristics, and attributes of that system:* The groups then prioritized their ideas, characteristics, and attributes. Following the retreat, nominal group and lateral thinking ideas were aggregated and given to each group member. Using the Delphi technique, based on the work of Delbecq, Van de Ven, and Gustafsen,[2] each person rated the importance of every idea for improving patient care on a scale of one to five. Mean scores were presented at a SPT meeting, and group members were given time to advocate for an idea they supported. This gave priority to five ideas that were moved forward to stage five. The ideas, along with the rankings and comments, were included in a summary report with the data collected from key stakeholders during the first stage. Inputs from stages one through four became the basis for identifying innovations to meet the desired delivery system requirements.

5. *Assessing stakeholder response to the desired delivery system:* Finally, the prioritized ideas were presented to more than 20 stakeholder groups institutionwide, including the medical board and PAC. These groups served to clarify the ideas, assess the extent of enthusiasm for change, and identify potential barriers to implementation. As George Belsey, former executive director and project codirector, indicates: "It was an opportunity to recommit to our mission and core values by identifying the gaps in what UH is providing compared to what is desired to serve the health care needs of the community."

6. *Developing prioritized ideas into action plans and implementable interventions:* In this final stage, task force groups involving more than 50 additional stakeholders, including physicians, managers, staff nurses, and other grass-roots staff, convened to clarify the top five ideas and identify:
   - Specific characteristics of the ideas
   - Measurable objectives for the ideas

- Specific activities or phases of implementation
- Implications for education and training
- Resources necessary to develop, implement, and evaluate the ideas
- Mechanisms to evaluate the impact of the ideas
- Stakeholders who would be affected by the ideas
- Issues related to implementation within the present organizational structure

• Three Programs That Evolved from the Process

The strategic planning process initially began with the objective of redesigning patient services to provide high-quality, cost-effective care across the continuum of service and to improve the supply and utilization of professional resources. Three innovative programs resulted from this process:

1. Restructured patient services
2. Multidisciplinary apprentice programs
3. Patient-centered services

Restructured Patient Services

Patient services were restructured through customized interdisciplinary patient service teams to coordinate care across care settings. This program is referred to as Service Teams with Appropriate Resources or STARs. When new STARs are formed, it is said, "A star is born."

Current Reality

UH is a traditional, functional hierarchy with departments organized by the specialized work of a given discipline. The medical staff is a separate hierarchy as part of the School of Medicine. The structure meets the needs of departments and disciplines, but does not effectively meet clinical efficiencies based on a patient-centered model. It does not allow for consistent and constant patterns of communication and collaboration. The boundaries dividing disciplines such as medicine, nursing, social work, and service areas (including inpatient care, outpatient care, home care, and alternative care) create barriers and issues for patients, their families, and caregivers. For example, patients and their families encounter numerous caregivers and often do not see the same caregiver throughout their inpatient stay. Caregivers spend an enormous amount of time attempting to collaborate and coordinate care. Balancing department needs with patient care clinical needs results in fragmented patient care that may not meet individual needs of the patient and family. The project staff indicates that "lack of coordination can result in an extra day of stay for the patient or redundant procedures such as laboratory and X ray." These inefficiencies create cost and quality concerns for patients, families, caregivers, and the hospital, including operational concerns and satisfaction issues.

The Desired Outcome, or Vision

The desired outcome is a system of patient care that crosses boundaries of geography and time and provides a consistent team of caregivers working collaboratively. The team would plan, coordinate, and implement care for the patient and family achieving agreed-upon quality outcomes. This vision led to restructuring clinical services by developing customized patient service teams with appropriate resources, or STARs. As Evelyn Hartigan, associate administrator for patient care services and project codirector, puts it: "STARs have responsibility and accountability for both the quality and cost of patient care."

The *STAR* is the basic organizational unit for delivery of patient and family services. It is a hospital-based group of interdisciplinary caregivers that follows patient care from the point of admission—emergency department, clinic, or physician office referral—through critical care and other inpatient services and then to home or an extended care facility. Each STAR is uniquely designed by multiple disciplines working together to best meet the needs of a specific group of patients throughout that continuum of service (as shown in figure 10-4), and each is coordinated by a nurse patient care coordinator (PCC). Cheryl Kinnear, STAR program manager, states that:

> Team membership is customized to the service needs of the patient group with a physician and nurse as consistent members. For example, [the] neuro-oncology STAR core team includes the neurosurgeon; a neuro-oncologist and fellow; a social worker; a pharmacist; physical, occupational, and speech therapists; a clinical dietitian; a representative from the managed care office; a home care nurse; and a RN from the neuroscience unit and ambulatory clinic. The neuro-oncology administrative secretary and support staff also have a role, along with consultive staff.

A STAR is "born" from an existing service after data review, including diagnosis-related groups, length of stay (LOS), census, demographic characteristics, acuity, common patient needs, and frequently used resources. Patient populations are clustered into groups with similar needs. Service location is considered in the selection of team members which include core (consistent), consultative (occasional), and supportive representatives. Once a STAR is formed, members convene to carry forward the planning and implementation processes. They determine relationships (including work and roles), team norms, the communication system, data collection, patient care outcomes, and other logistics pertinent to working together. STARs are being

Figure 10-4. Customized Patient Care

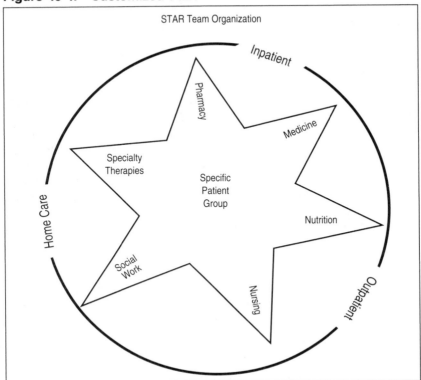

Source: University Hospital's Program to Improve Patient Care, University of Utah, Salt Lake City.

piloted in the neuroscience and rehabilitation services. The success of the pilots will determine whether the model will be expanded to other services such as obstetrics, orthopedics, and oncology.

Thus far, a number of improvements in quality of care have been demonstrated. These include:

- Improved coordination of care decisions resulting in less duplication of laboratory testing and X rays
- Improved therapy planning resulting in decreased delays
- Improved discharge planning resulting in discharge plans initiated during the admission process, at times decreasing LOS and readmission rates, including improved appropriate utilization of emergency services
- Initiated prehospital patient care preparation resulting in improved understanding and satisfaction by the patients and their families about what to expect
- Improved collaboration, respect, and trust among caregivers

- Increased understanding of what each STAR team member contributes to the outcome of patient care

Other operational improvements resulting from improved communication and more specific data collection are resulting in organizational efficiencies. Many are value added but difficult to quantify, such as improved satisfaction with the quality of work life by stakeholders participating in STAR formation and implementation.

The restructuring of patient services influenced UH to consider a modified matrix organization. A matrix organization works best when team organization is superimposed on a functional hierarchy. "Vertical coordination occurs as each department maintains its functional operations," explains Beck. "Horizontal coordination occurs through the direct interaction of the STAR members who perform the clinical work of patient care." In a pure matrix organization, two formal lines of authority exist. The modified matrix preserves the decision-making process of the existing chain of command and maintains reporting relationships of staff to one manager. The standard of practice for a given discipline resides with the functional department. The matrix organization emphasizes increased flexibility and participation in decision making by levels of staff throughout the hospital. It supports enhanced autonomy for the STARs, yet provides the necessary structure and direction from top leadership.

Multidisciplinary Apprentice Programs

Multidisciplinary apprentice programs (MAPs) are designed to provide a flexible and versatile assistant health care worker who will have an opportunity to become a health professional. The objectives of MAP are to: (1) Improve utilization by use of assistant workers, and (2) Increase supply of health professionals and allied workers.

Current Reality

The SPT facilitated the nursing practice department (NPD) to recognize that many professionals are facing shortages or distribution issues. Vacancy rates for allied health workers, including respiratory therapists (RTs) and physical therapists (PTs), average greater than 10 percent nationally. Health professionals are needed in great numbers for ambulatory, prevention, wellness, and home care services. Health care cost reforms are requiring redesign of work and roles to utilize appropriately RNs and other health care professionals. In preparing for the type of work force needed now and in the future, and to reduce work force cost while maintaining quality of care and services provided by the appropriate caregiver, UH renewed its interest in the support worker.

Numerous new models such as nurse extenders, unit assistants, dyads, and partners in practice emerged in an attempt to provide nurses with support for direct and indirect patient care. Although position combining and cross-training increase worker productivity, particularly in hospital inpatient and outpatient settings, UH leaders felt these models did not systematically consider where the work force will be needed in the future and what type of worker will be required in different care settings. In 1989, few nonlicensed support personnel were employed in the NPD. Numerous other departments were using support personnel, each trained and specialized to one particular department, to carry out support tasks relating only to that department. There were 46 support level job descriptions. Historically, these positions had a high turnover rate with associated costs for recruitment and training.

Desired Outcome, or Vision

The multidisciplinary apprentice program emerged from the strategic planning process. The multidisciplinary apprentice program is designed to prepare a flexible and versatile technical health care worker. It offers potential for workers, depending on aptitude and interest, to progress via formal academic preparation to the level of health care professional. In addition to meeting the initial need for increasing the support work force, it also considers future work force needs.

The multidisciplinary apprentice program provides in-house cross-training for entry-level staff in indirect and direct patient care. The basic training consists of medical terminology, interpersonal and human relation skills, and nursing assistant curricula developed by the Utah State Board of Education. Cross-training includes selected skills performed by a health unit coordinator (formerly called unit secretary), a respiratory therapy aide, and a physical therapy assistant. Apprentices receive guidance and counseling toward either a professional career such as nursing, physical therapy, or pharmacy, or a technical career such as respiratory technician or X-ray technician. Apprentices have formal and informal opportunities to explore potential career tracks through lectures, observational experiences, and interactions with health care professionals.

Over time, apprentices progress through four levels of learning. (See figure 10-5.) In level 1, the apprentice has six months to learn to perform indirect and direct patient care. The competency-based course involves two class days per week. The other three days are spent applying new skills by working in a predetermined patient care area. Apprentices are assigned to both inpatient and ambulatory care, where they assist health professionals in activities that do not require direct patient contact. Cross-training includes activities such as order transcription, telephone skills, and patient scheduling for procedures performed by the health unit coordinator. As they begin to master skills in direct care, each apprentice works with an RN care partner

Figure 10-5. Multidisciplinary Apprentice Program Cross-Training and Career Tracks

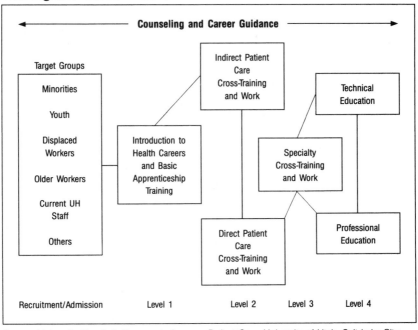

Source: University Hospital's Program to Improve Patient Care, University of Utah, Salt Lake City.

who has been recruited as a volunteer from the nursing staff. Apprentices and RNs work the same shift schedule to facilitate their partnership, and the RN delegates the specific tasks the apprentice is to perform for each patient.

After passing the state certification examination for certified nursing assistants, apprentices advance to level 2. They continue to work full-time in assigned patient care areas, but now are assigned to a variety of RN partners, increasing the opportunity for on-the-job learning. Progression to level 3 occurs once the apprentice has made a career decision and prerequisite courses are initiated. After the apprentice has completed the requirements for level 3, he or she either applies for an available support worker position in an area compatible with training, such as physical therapy or home care, or advances to one of several newly developed positions involving additional skills and cross-training. For example, a cross-trained position is being developed in the perioperative setting. It will combine the technical skills of surgical processing, the operating room, and the postanesthesia care unit. Apprentices work in these positions as they complete prerequisite study and apply for admission into a formal educational program. Upon acceptance, they progress to level 4. As health professionals or technical students, they continue to work at the hospital with the support of flexible scheduling and tuition reimbursement.

A comprehensive recruitment plan for MAP includes relationships with community organizations in touch with desired target populations. MAP targeted recruitment to persons who traditionally did not enter health professions: youth, minorities, dislocated and displaced workers, and older workers. Current hospital employees in entry-level positions such as linen, nutrition care, and environmental services were encouraged to apply. The first recruitment effort was a great success with a class of 14 apprentices drawn from more than 120 applicants. All target groups were represented in the applicant pool and class. Completing three years of demonstration, MAP will become institutionalized as a part of human resource functions.

Patient-Centered Services

Patient-centered services are intended to provide patients and their families with tools to facilitate their involvement in decision making.

The Vision

The SPT wanted to distinguish the quality of health care from the quality of service. It idealized a vision to provide services based on patient needs. The team wanted patients and families to know what to expect and to play a role in care decisions. Jackie Smith, project manager, patient-centered services, explains:

> Patients and their families expressed a desire during information-gathering forums to receive more information about what they could expect before coming to the hospital and while they were in the hospital. They expressed a desire to be active participants in decision making about their care.

Current Reality

Patient and family satisfaction with service is dependent on their expectations and perceptions of service. As the project team indicates, "Setting clear expectations allows the patient and family to anticipate the experience of hospitalization with less fear of the unknown." When patient expectations are known, their confirmation or lack of confirmation can be assessed by the caregiver based on the patient's perception of the actual service received. When there is agreement between what is expected and what is perceived, patient satisfaction increases.

Desired Outcome

Patient-centered services are intended to strengthen the quality of service through the notion that service is driven by patient needs rather than institutional needs. The Service Expectation Program and the "U" CHOOSE Program are examples of the patient-centered philosophy.

The Service Expectation Program is designed to meet patient expectations prior to or at the time of admission through a videotape (titled *First Impressions*) and supplementary written materials. The videotape is modular in format, and its script was reviewed for content and accuracy by key hospital stakeholders, including patients. An indexing system allows patients and their families to selectively view specific modules, which generally are less than 15 minutes in length. Modules include: a welcome and introduction to the hospital, the admitting process, patient room orientation, daily hospital routine, meals, available amenities, the health care team, pastoral care, the billing practice, and the discharge planning process. The modular format also allows for customized information. For example, the video can be combined with a preoperative video for surgical patients. Other options in the design stage are for different types of admissions — for example, at home prior to admission, in the clinic or physician office, and in the admitting area or patient room at the time of admission.

Supplementary written materials included with the video provide various phone numbers of importance to the patient, including the physician's number. Reference materials can be customized, for example, to include a list of STAR team members. The materials are produced in a modular fashion using insert cards so that a packet can be assembled based on individual patient needs.

The "U" CHOOSE Program extends the concept of patient-centered service beyond giving information to allowing patients and their families to become involved in care decisions. It offers actual choices about services and provides opportunities to personalize the hospital stay. Choices for personalizing service are designed in four categories: (1) personal hygiene and comfort (for example, time for bathing); (2) prescribed care (for example, self-medication); (3) dietary and nutrition (number of meals per day); and (4) discharge planning (for example, referral for home care). Amenities or specialized services such as a professional massage will be made available at an additional charge. This program is intended to enhance patient control and autonomy, thereby promoting family and patient involvement in decisions about their needs and preparing them for self-care. Usually the patient and caregiver work together to make choices in customizing services.

A phase-in approach for patient-centered services is adapted to identify and discuss many legal, ethical, financial, and human resource utilization concerns. Phase I involves establishing 16 formalized methods to inform patients about services and options currently available. Expansion of services and options involving controversial legal, ethical, and operational issues will follow in later phases. The Division of Medical Ethics is involved in guiding analysis of these issues. State-of-the-art interactive television and other media are being explored to provide service options.

• Difficulties in Developing an Integrated Process

Despite the benefits of this integrated approach, a number of difficulties also emerged. Some of these were:

- Transitioning from recommendations to implementation
- Defining SPT authority because decision-making and follow-through accountability resided with the existing hospital groups
- Passing the decision process between structures rather than dealing with it directly
- Defining relationships between traditional leaders and grass-roots stake-holders, particularly between directors and staff who are not members of the same department

Gilmore confirms these dilemmas in his work on institutionalizing transformations.[3] A process of this nature often begins enthusiastically for a variety of reasons, including:

- People are enabled to articulate feelings and think about personal and organizational purpose.
- Coalitions are mobilized between departments.
- Responsibility is shared by everyone.
- Experimentation, creativity, and imagination are encouraged.
- Resulting actions are for improved patient care services.

Later, people begin to realize that permissiveness or empowerment means different things to different people. They are required to regroup to learn about each other and progress from discussions to dialogue, from cooperation to collaboration, and from independence or codependence to interdependence. They require tools and methods for learning new behaviors and practices. Participants may require assurance that resources will be available. Sensitivity and sensibility are required by leadership and a commitment that demonstrates overt involvement and not merely talk. These dilemmas will lessen as parallel structures created for innovations become institutionalized and formal communication systems are established between the new aspects of the structure and the existing chain of command.

References

1. De Bono, E. *Lateral Thinking: Creativity Step by Step.* New York City: Harper and Row, 1970.
2. Delbecq, A. L., Van de Ven, A. H., and Gustafsen, D. H. *Group Techniques and Program Planning: A Guide to Nominal Group Technique and Delphi Process.* Glenview, IL: Scott Foresman, 1975.
3. Gilmore, T. N. Dilemmas of institutionalizing transformations. SHNP education program, Orlando, FL, Sept. 1993.

• Appendix. Listening to the Language of Patients

The University of Utah Hospital (UH) conducted several patient focus groups as part of its strategic planning process. It also used these groups to test concepts of the three innovative outcomes of UH's Program to Improve Patient Care. UH chose to use focus group discussions because they provide a particularly useful way to obtain input and understand the patient perspective in the patient's own language.

The "language of patients" that follows consists of comments from patients who participated in three focus groups held at the hospital in December 1991. The groups consisted of both inpatients and outpatients from the neuroscience and rehabilitation services. The overall goal of their discussions was threefold: to learn about patient expectations of service, to obtain patient opinions, and to identify patient perceptions on ways to improve care delivery. Suggestions were sought on ways to coordinate care, increase satisfaction levels, utilize care teams, and give patients more control over their hospital stays. Several major themes emerged from the group discussions, which are presented below in the patients' own words.

"Desire to Be Treated Courteously and with Respect"

Patients did not like being "talked down to." They appreciated being called by correct (or preferred) titles (for example, Mr., Mrs., or Dr.) and being acknowledged as a person with choices and preferences. One patient said: "I was really impressed with some people as they came up and said 'What's your name or what would you like me to call you.'" Patients did not want to be treated impersonally, for example, "like an object" or a "research subject" or "like you're something they find in a lecture hall." They expressed preferences for caregivers who were kind, considerate, and willing to make others

---

This appendix was prepared by Jackie A. Smith, PhD, University Hospital/University of Utah; Debra L. Scammon, University of Utah; and Susan Beck, RN, PhD, University Hospital/ University of Utah, Salt Lake City.

happy and comfortable. They appreciated providers who used positive reinforcement rather than authoritative or dictating commands. They felt that a hospital centered on the patient would have caregivers who put their hearts into care, as well as their skill and knowledge. Comments reflective of their feelings include:

- "Nurses should be like a caring family . . . they are your buddies."
- "I like to be treated with understanding."
- "I would like nurses to be my friend."
- "I get along with all of my nurses . . . they are all friendly."
- "Because I'm caring, I need someone with me who will work with me."
- "I want a therapist to push me — to make me work for it. Not to be hard-headed and mean, but to be my friend."
- "I guess I enjoyed him [the nurse] so much because he didn't push me around. He wasn't tough, he didn't get mad at me, no matter what I did. He didn't put me down. He was kind, considerate. When you're in the hospital in pain, kindness and consideration mean a great deal."

"Need More Information and Communication"

Focus group participants in all three groups wanted more information on hospital activities, treatment alternatives and plans, what to expect during their hospital stays, and how to communicate concerns to the staff. One patient noted: "I didn't know what to expect. I didn't know if I was going to have a say."

Additionally, patients who participated in the focus groups clearly expressed the desire to have information provided in language and terminology they understood. As one patient who had been diagnosed with a brain tumor indicated: "A lot of doctors expect patients are automatically going to know what they are talking about, because to them, it's such a common topic or subject or term. That causes lack of understanding by the patient."

Other group participants indicated:

- "I want to know exactly what the situation is. I'm not a medical person. I don't know all the big words and everything, but I want to know what the situation is."
- "I need therapists to be able to explain why they are doing a certain thing, because I've had some times where I've had a therapist sit there and tell me to do something and I'm just kind of like asking, 'Why am I doing this? Would you tell me what I'm doing this for?'"
- "When doctors communicate, they use long terms that patients don't understand. They need to use terms that everyone can understand, real English."
- "Inform us before changes; give us a voice of concern."

Focus group participants often expressed the desire for more information on their hospital experience and the care they were to receive. They expressed concern about not knowing what to expect or ask for and what their limits of control were. Participants provided a long list of items to include in the *First Impressions* video and resource packet. They also readily promoted the idea of receiving this information before a hospital stay, whenever possible. Specifically, they were looking for information on: how to call the hospital, parking, insurance, the admitting process, what to wear in the hospital, what to bring or not to bring, hospital rooms, daily activities, shift changes, caregivers, and the billing system.

Participants also felt that it was important to prepare the family for a patient's hospital stay. Family involvement was viewed as extremely important in situations where patients are brought to the hospital through the emergency department or are too ill to be able to comprehend information regarding their care.

One of the disappointments for some of the focus group participants is not being informed about treatment plans and alternatives. In referring to diagnostic tests, one patient exclaimed: "I've never had one explained to me yet." Repeatedly, focus group participants indicate that they wanted to know more about their treatment plans, their progress, and when they could expect reports. They recognized that medical conditions sometimes make it difficult for them to remember things they are told, and appreciate reminders and information reinforcement. "A nurse was absolutely in control of everything. He also would talk to me, tell me about what happened."

One group participant wanted more information on her treatment alternatives and spent a lot of time in the library "trying to figure out what my options were and how successful the various options were." For this patient, "Having somebody from the hospital [who] basically broke down the research into layman terms and had a sheet that described the various options, where the state of research is on these things in layman terms, and how success[ful] they might have been, might have been a very useful thing to do."

Patients also desire a mechanism through which direct, confidential feedback about their care could be provided without reprisal. Or as patients expressed it: "When you are between life and death, you don't want to say too much because they might turn the switch off. Sometimes its hard to express concerns or complaints because you don't want to open a can of worms and end up in a big mess." Another patient reported: "It's hard to be assertive."

• "Increased Coordination Is Helpful"

The concept of coordination within the hospital also was explored with focus group participants. The moderator of the groups specifically asked patients where and when they had experienced coordination problems and if they had suggestions to remedy some of their concerns. The idea of having a patient care coordinator help with these issues was also proposed to the groups. Many patients replied: "If I had the nurse that I contact now and who I contacted when I was in chemotherapy come up and visit me or someone was reporting to her, I would have felt a lot better about the time I spent in the hospital." Clearly, they felt that someone should be assigned to communicate: "We have ward clerks and charge nurses, so there should be someone that's in charge of communicating information."

Participants reported paperwork duplication, lack of communication among providers, and in some cases a lack of coordination and communication overall. One specific area cited for improvement was that of reducing repetitive form completion. As one group participant put it: "Every time you move from one room to another, you have to fill out the same paperwork." Another area for improvement was coordination with outpatient physicians: "There are too many doctors and they're not all communicating with each other."

One participant illustrated patient sensitivity to the nurses' lack of coordination. Her sensitivity was heightened by her medical condition. She said: "Every nurse that is on this floor should be able to give meds. There are night nurses that cannot give you any meds; they have to go find another nurse to give you your meds — then you wait 20 minutes — like you're going to suffer pain . . . there is a long 45 minutes between shift changes." Another patient indicated: "I think there should be a facilitator when the students come in to make it clear to the patient as to who these people are. They've made some attempt at this already. I'm not saying they just barge into the door and start stabbing and poking, that's not it. Just the same, I think there should be a little more organization there. We're here and if you don't want us here, we'll go away or we'll come back or something. A little more gentle bedside manner."

Patients often used the word *facilitator* when referring to having someone to "facilitate" patient care with other health care providers and to assist with discharge planning. A consistent facilitator is viewed as a "troubleshooter," "educator" (about hospital activities), "coordinator," "communicator," and "confidential advocate" to help the patient's stay go smoother and faster. This type of coordination was viewed by one patient as "a strong support system that encourages the patient to come out of themselves and to try harder." One patient summarized the coordination of care that patients want this way: "I think it needs to be like this: that the center needs to be, instead of department centralized, it ought to be patient centralized. Be concerned about each patient and whatever is best for that patient."

Patients also desired better coordination in the admitting process. They wanted to see admitting streamlined with files available on patients who come to the hospital often. One suggestion involved having a computerized system to help coordinate room availability and to decrease waiting time. Long waiting times in several areas of the hospital, without being told the reason for the delay, are a source of frustration for patients.

• "Desire for More Control and Choices"

Participants (particularly those in rehabilitation) wanted to go to the cafeteria or snack bar for meals, participate in giving their own medications, have library services with audio capabilities, have more television options, have more food choices, and have choices regarding personal items such as shampoos and soaps. They wanted more control over timing of events such as choosing when to get up, shower, go to bed, and turn out the lights.

In exploring desired options, the facilitator used the phrase "menu of choices." Participants were confused; they thought of this as a food menu. Because of this confusion, prior to implementation of the options program, the term was replaced with "U" Choose.

• Conclusion

The inpatients and outpatients who participated in the three focus groups provided myriad suggestions for improving patient care at University Hospital. The groups clearly stated their expectations and ideas for program development and refinement. The information has proved useful in development of the STARs program along with specific patient-centered service activities such as *First Impressions,* "U" Choose, and customer service training.

Overall participants were pleased with the care they receive at UH, and expressed appreciation for being able to participate in the focus groups and provide input. The language of patients heard during these group discussions demonstrates the value of patient input for program planning as well as for improving existing services.

Chapter 11 _____

Providence Portland Medical Center

"A style of decision making focused on asking people how can we solve the problem together" is the way that Colleen Burch, assistant head nurse, neurology, urology, ENT, gynecology, and pediatrics, characterizes the change in culture at Providence Portland Medical Center (PPMC), in Portland, Oregon. The change is based on a model for shared decision making that will achieve shared understanding. Involvement in decision making stimulates staff energy and momentum to make the organization's vision real and to get the organization where it wants to be. According to Burch, "Those involved are now more likely to think through who is affected by the decision, so they are invited to be at the table for discussion and decision making. This process of shared decision making helps participants break out of their usual way of thinking." This chapter describes the model that PPMC designed to change its culture and achieve its vision.

• The PPMC Model

The model used at PPMC is a generative process beginning with leadership. The other components of the model, illustrated in figure 11-1, are shared decision making, shared understanding, and organizational learning and adaptability.

Leadership

Leadership creates the environment for shared decision making (SDM) through the formation of "structures." At PPMC, these structures are composed of

Chapter 11 was prepared by Marie J. Driever, RN, PhD, coproject director, Redesign and Improvement for Patient Care Delivery, Providence Portland Medical Center, Portland, Oregon. Mary Schoessler, RN, MS, assistant director, nursing education, Providence Portland Medical Center, is acknowledged for her valuable review and critique of this chapter.

Figure 11-1.   The PPMC Model

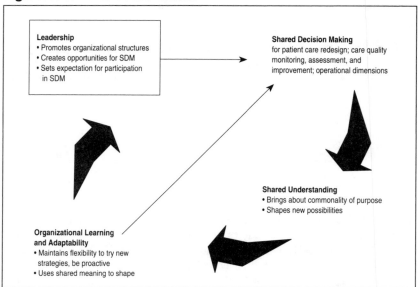

Source: Redesign and Improvement for Patient Care Delivery, Providence Portland Medical Center, Portland, Oregon.

interdisciplinary caregivers at various levels of the organization, from staff to administration. Through its Redesign and Improvement of Care Delivery project (discussed later in this chapter), PPMC has experimented with ways to organize SDM structures as teams and councils so that there are mechanisms for joint decision making at the unit, middle, and executive levels of the organization. The councils create the environment for SDM by framing the issues that require decisions. For example, unit-level SDM councils have given impetus for the redesign of the nurse role. Bert Sperry, nurse manager, respiratory and medical units, explains:

> SDM channeled the self-directed energy of the staff to make role changes happen through deciding the issues needing to be addressed, redefining the role of the primary nurse, and then providing the support for the role to happen. . . . This joint working through of decisions truly create a lasting change.

Unit-based SDM councils also create the new and necessary modes of communication required to work with other disciplines in this redesign effort.

For leadership to be effective, requirements for SDM must be viewed from three leadership perspectives: administrative, managerial, and staff. (See figure 11-2.) Austinson explains these requirements:

These requirements help to define certain leader characteristics. Leaders must temper results desired with ground-level ownership of the process of achieving results; provide constant recognition of efforts through acknowledging what people are doing, why they are doing it, how far they have come, and how their efforts relate to the whole. Leadership also involves serving as an educator using coaching and mentoring strategies and structuring constant discussion about the desirability of having the kind of culture that values and therefore actively supports shared decision making.

Leadership also must cultivate sensitivity to "see" the numerous situations that constitute opportunities for SDM by these structures at all levels of the organization and to set expectations for staff participation.

Shared Decision Making

SDM functions at various levels of the organization and serves to accomplish several purposes. These include the redesign of patient care delivery, development of indicators for monitoring achievement of ongoing improvement in the quality of care provided, and management of day-to-day operations issues, including implementation of changing technology and use of resources.

Figure 11-2. Requirements for SDM from Three Leadership Perspectives

Administrative	Managerial	Staff
• Administrative attitude and willingness to believe and trust; believe people can be trusted to do high-quality work; let go so that people can create something; an ability to tolerate ambiguity.	• Managers must create environment to promote staff self-direction; support SDM structures and new models of communication.	• Staff must be willing to accept invitation to participate, acknowledge feelings engendered by change, take ownership of the change effects inherent in SDM.
• To make SDM work, set and communicate vision, provide general parameters to guide people's work, have check points to monitor progress and results.	• To make SDM work, managers and staff together must decide issues to be changed.	• To make SDM work, reach out to management and staff involved in decision to be made, listen to why change is needed, treat each other with respect, care about what is said; be willing to use information to ask questions and see situation differently.

SDM is at the heart of the culture change at PPMC. It incorporates an expectation of participation in decision making by staff at all levels of the organization and a sense of inclusiveness to make the decision-making process work. Arlene Austinson, assistant administrator, nursing and patient care, explains that the sense of inclusiveness "more and more frequently results in inviting staff from across care delivery settings—that is, home health, the payer or insurance component of the system, and not just those from within the hospital—to focus on the patient's longitudinal care needs."

Using SDM, managers and staff together provide examples of setting expectations for participation in decision making, and the staff response to trusting these expectations is now part of the changed culture at PPMC. "In one instance," indicates Burch, "decision making by one unit staff helped their manager decrease staff resources due to budget constraints." In a broader arena, the administration invited a unit to help determine how another unit's patient population and staff could be merged so that one unit could be closed due to a decrease in patient census. Burch cites another example: "I see more opportunities for involvement by staff in decision making such as the identification and organization of resources to support staff education for major information system technology changes." Now staff are invited to be part of the decisions on how to provide staff coverage during initial implementation, the kind and amount of education required, and the tools and other resources necessary to make introduction of major changes in the information system successful.

Even with the council structures, staff members still need to be invited consistently to participate in SDM. This is very important because their expectation of inclusion and participation is necessary for gaining their trust in (1) the process and (2) their role in the process. Additionally, they must believe that their participation will be valued and their opinions listened to. Consistently inviting staff participation in SDM, particularly when tough decisions have to be made, builds trust and a sense of security that will enable them to make decisions with confidence and come to believe that decisions made by a group are better than those made by individuals. Inclusion also fosters staff awareness of who constitutes the relevant stakeholders to be invited; in other words, staff become more conscious of who needs to be at the table when decisions must be made. Burch summarizes: "The invitation to participate acknowledges the changes that are the focus of decision making and that these changes affect staff. Staff acceptance of the invitation creates the beginning ownership of the changes that are and must be made."

For those engaged in and committed to the SDM process, a reward system must be in place that involves creative options for continuing professional development. For example, in addition to formal recognition and promotion, the organization might offer assistance to those staff members who wish to publish.

Shared Understanding

The concept of shared understanding, which is essential to the SDM model, is derived from the work of Morgan.[1,2] *Shared understanding* is the bringing together of people with diverse perspectives to work on a common endeavor and thus to find shared meaning of the situation. The concept involves being able to tolerate differences, because it does not command total agreement. Shared understanding also involves the joint shaping of new possibilities in terms of how to implement an organization's vision, purposes, and goals. Constant change creates the need for continual renewal of common understanding in order to assist and provide support and reinforcement for everyone to work toward agreed-upon goals.

Organizational Learning and Adaptability

The ability to use decision-making opportunities, not only to solve problems but also to bring about shared understanding, is at the core of organizational learning, which in turn promotes adaptability. *Adaptability* is the constant striving of individuals from all levels of the organization to learn together and to develop a common understanding of how to respond to new demands placed on the organization. Individual and team flexibility is manifested in a willingness to think about new ways of "seeing" opportunities to provide and improve care delivery. Organizational learning requires that people work through issues to arrive at joint decisions and engage in dialogue to create the meaning necessary for shared decision making. This in turn fosters an environment that promotes energy, momentum, and creativity.

• The Redesign and Improvement for Patient Care Delivery Project

The Redesign and Improvement for Patient Care Delivery project is an integration of PPMC's patient care delivery redesign and quality improvement initiatives. PPMC used a trajectory model to develop a new and improved care delivery system that is continuous, flexible, and responsive to what the patient requires. The focus of the work is to produce patient care outcomes that guide the design for improvements across the continuum of care. Learning is the essence of restructuring because it unites individual, group, and organizational efforts to transform mind-sets and generate needed changes. Institutionwide restructuring has focused on shared decision making, systems of care delivery, and relationships. This has resulted in:

- Strengthened continuity of care for patients across all care settings
- Improved collaborative relationships among payers, providers, and caregivers

- Redefined roles for caregivers
- Rethinking of resource allocation, including in the provision of care outside the hospital and across the Sister of Providence Health System
- Stimulation of the use of technology in care delivery and for redesign and improvement endeavors

The project is influencing care delivery within the Oregon region of the Sisters of Providence Health System through its approach, satisfaction with staff involvement, and positive patient care outcomes.

References

1. Morgan, G. _Imaginization: The Art of Creative Management._ Newbury Park, CA: Sage Publications, 1993.

2. Morgan, G. _Personal Communication._ Newbury Park, CA: Sage Publications, 1995.

Chapter 12

Health BOND

In the late 1980s, Kathryn Schweer, former dean of Mankato State University (MSU) School of Nursing, and Annette McBeth, vice-president, Immanuel-St. Joseph's Hospital, posed the question: "What should nursing education and the health care system be like as we move into the 21st century?" The existing system offered many inequities and few, if any, linkages between service organizations in south central Minnesota and local educational institutions. Thus, Schweer and McBeth initiated a visioning process based on shared values and shared beliefs about high-quality health status and ways in which nursing education could influence improved health care delivery. Their visioning was based on professional commitment to an integrated regional health care system in which nursing education would play a significant role. This commitment required a change in attitude on the part of both service and education leaders, as well as in the relationship between the institutions. To initiate the change, they defined two shared goals: (1) to provide education for nurses and enhance their ability to improve the health status of individuals and their families; and (2) to achieve improved access for health services in south central Minnesota for everyone, regardless of economic status. These shared goals were the foundation for their SHNP project — Health BOND (Building Opportunities and New Directions). This chapter describes the Health BOND project and its shared governance model.

• A Partnership Model: Health BOND

Health BOND is an informal, voluntary consortium made up of three hospitals — Immanuel-St. Joseph's Hospital, Arlington Municipal Hospital,

Chapter 12 was prepared by Health BOND partners Annette McBeth, RN, MS, vice-president, Immanuel St. Joseph's Hospital, Mankato, Minnesota; Kathryn Schweer, RN, PhD, former dean of Mankato State University School of Nursing, Mankato, Minnesota; and Sharon Aadalen, project director, Health BOND Consortium, Mankato, Minnesota.

and Waseca Area Memorial Hospital—and two educational institutions—Mankato State University Technical College (renamed South Central Technical College) and Mankato State University. It represents a partnership between service and education, and is built on the principles of shared leadership and shared values.

The Starting Point

Ackoff's interactive planning model presented during the 1989 SHNP educational session set the tone for rethinking, conversation, and new insights among Health BOND executive leaders, physician and trustee representatives, and project staff.[1] He presented this situation: "You have just received news that your respective hospitals have burned down. How would you go about redesigning and rebuilding them?" To expand on this scenario, he narrated an event that occurred in the telephone industry. In the 1970s, the CEO of Bell Telephone posed a similar problem to key employees: "What would you do if the entire telephone system went down? How would you go about redesigning and rebuilding it?" His intention was to challenge employees to think differently and to come up with innovations in an industry in which nothing new had surfaced since the 1960s. His challenge produced a variety of innovations, including FAX, visual communication, voice mail, touch tone dialing, portable phones, and cellular phones. These innovations were developed on the premise of creating "the ideal communication system." Realizing the importance of this way of thinking, consortium leaders were motivated to design the ideal health care delivery system for south central Minnesota.

As a starting point for redesigning the regional health care system, each hospital team (consisting of executives, trustee and physician representatives, project staff, managers, and caregivers) considered two situations:

1. You are the patient coming into the hospital: "What would you like as your ideal way to receive care?"
2. You have been assigned to rebuild this hospital and redesign the nursing education system at MSU and South Central Technical College: "How would you deliver health care maintaining quality health care and cost efficiencies, and how would you design the education system to meet the work force needs?"

The Outcomes

Three themes emerged from the collaborative working sessions. These were:

1. Redesigned health care services will provide high-quality, cost-effective patient- and family-centered care.

2. Redesigned health care services are integrated regionally through service and education partnerships.
3. Consortium organizations are the providers and employers of choice for people we serve in the region.

These themes continue to be key elements in the shared vision statement and foundation of Health BOND.

As the partnership evolved and trust deepened, consortium members identified shared objectives to guide them in realizing their vision. These objectives are:

• To provide leadership through an interactive planning process for developing a regional health care system responsive to rural consumers
• To develop indicators to measure improvement in the quality and cost-effectiveness of care and service throughout the redesign process
• To promote cultural change among members of the health care team to facilitate continuous quality improvement
• To improve coordination of services promoting a continuum of patient- and family-centered health care
• To integrate a regional network of services and education providers

Health BOND leaders agree that proactive participation, commitment to the vision, and trust in each other are the hallmarks of creating a more desirable health care delivery system for their region. To ensure meaningful participation and contribution by all stakeholders, Health BOND designed and implemented a three-day education and training session entitled Leaders Empower Staff, and developed an integrated decentralized infrastructure to support and ensure their partnership agreement. The infrastructure is designed as an interorganizational shared governance model.

The Shared Governance Model

The shared governance model promotes the sharing of resources, leadership development, coordinated action, and innovative work groups across consortium member institutions for the purpose of regional health care improvements. Its design is circular, with the executive committee and coordinating council at the core of the circle and four satellite standing committees. (See figure 12-1.) Sharon Aadalen, consortium project director for Health BOND, describes the model's organizational layers:

The executive committee and coordinating council are the core of the model. The executive committee has accountability for budget decisions and review and approval of interdisciplinary innovation. The coordinating council [composed of senior-level leadership from each of the member hospitals, faculty from the education partners, and project staff] has overall

Figure 12-1.   Shared Governance Structure

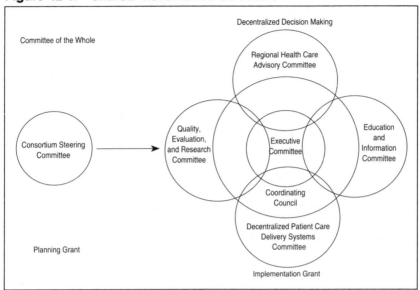

Source: Health Bond: Service and Education Partnership in South Central Minnesota.

accountability for Health BOND, and provides the leadership for developing a regional health care system responsive to rural consumers. The next
organizational layer consists of standing committees linked together and
interacting with the core governing bodies. The standing committees develop indicators, identify data sources and report types, define accountable
parties, and describe processes for providing feedback to stakeholders
related to achievement of stated objectives. . . . The circular, interlinking design symbolizes the integration of strategies which are the work of
the standing committees. The shared governance structure promotes
representation from all member partners and from the community.

Committee membership is based on the following guidelines:

- Individuals with skills to implement the following functions: administration, care providers (nurses, physicians, and other professionals),
  information systems, finances, human resources, service and academic
  education, patient care evaluation, research and statistics, and corporate business
- Leaders with ability and organizational talent to influence shifts in
  thinking from bureaucratic structures to those that support continuum
  of care frameworks for providing patient services
- Regional and community representatives, including businesses, service agencies, public health, and county and regional officials, along
  with organizational partners

The Standing Committees

The four standing committees in the shared governance model are the Regional Health Care Committee, the Decentralized Patient Care Delivery Systems Committee, the Education and Information Committee, and the Quality, Evaluation, and Research Committee. Following is a breakdown of each committee's responsibilities:

Regional Health Care Committee

This committee is charged with assessing regional health care needs. These include:

- Customer requirements for service and quality of a specific service
- Evaluation processes to demonstrate utilization and effectiveness of services
- Vertical integration strategies across the continuum of care
- Strategic planning processes for consolidation and networking among providers and payers

The committee's assessment survey is coordinated by the Community Health Services Unit of the Minnesota Department of Health and the Region Nine Development Commission. Using the assessment data, underserved populations and many of the health care problems specific to the region are identified. Problems include transportation, nutrition for the elderly and shut-ins, wellness and prevention education, and service accessibility. Analysis of the data is a collaborative planning effort facilitated by the Region Nine Development Commission and Health BOND. This collaborative effort created a Rural Health Planning Conference for key community representatives (including politicians, commissioners, consumers, and health care providers) from the area. The purpose of the conference is to share the assessment data and to identify the next steps. The Region Nine Advisory Committee, representing participants from the conference, is an outgrowth of the conference along with a Region Nine Rural Health Profile prepared by Wendi Lindquist, an urban and regional studies graduate student at MSU. The profile is sponsored by the Region Nine Health Advisory Committee, South Central Minnesota Emergency Medical Services, the Region Nine Area Agency on Aging, and Medtronics, Inc.

Decentralized Patient Care Delivery Systems Committee

This committee focuses on how to facilitate services coordination on a continued basis versus providing episodic care embracing the principles of a primary nursing care delivery system. Models that address patient health concerns beyond the walls of acute care are examined and linkages are established with organizations experienced with case management methods. The committee is developing criteria and care plans for case-managing high-resource-utilization patient populations and clinical pathways for specific patient populations. Pathways and case management practices are developed collaboratively by hospital and educational partners, and are operationalized with modifications as appropriate by the individual institution.

Education and Information Committee

Recognizing the need for cultural change in the member hospitals, this committee analyzes and recommends modalities for innovation and continuous quality improvement. Its functions include:

- *Work satisfaction studies:* These were conducted in 1989 for RNs and in 1990 and 1993 for LPNs (the Stamps and Piedmont Tool[2]). The 1990 study, under the direction of Howard Miller, associate professor of management and industrial relations, MSU College of Business, set the baseline for all member hospitals. Studies are repeated every two years to measure the impact, process, and outcomes of overall employee work satisfaction. The findings show that work satisfaction improved significantly between 1989 and 1993.
- *Leaders Empower Staff education and training:* This leadership training program is offered to senior-level leaders, unit-level hospital staff, and education partners. It focuses on leadership skills and techniques such as communication strategies, interdisciplinary team building, conflict resolution, consensus building, project management, and evaluation methods. The training format uses active learning strategies in which members learn skills and techniques of empowerment and leadership. The skills are role-modeled in different leadership and problem-solving situations. Ongoing renewal sessions are included in institutional employee education and training programs.
- *Regional Continuing Health Care Education Council (ReCheck):* This council is responsible for ongoing assessment of educational and training needs of regional education and service providers. It determines how the consortium can prepare the work force of the future to meet continuum of care service needs of patients and their families in south central Minnesota.

Quality, Evaluation, and Research Committee

This committee is charged with developing and implementing a standard evaluation framework so as to measure quality of care and cost-effectiveness of service outcomes. It began by considering the question: "How do we know where we are going if we do not know where we started from?" By examining their shared vision and desired interventions, members are able to identify indicators demonstrating service effectiveness and cost efficiencies. They collect and report baseline data from which they measure progress by identifying the impact at any time during the planning and implementation stage of a new initiative or intervention.

Challenges to the Governance Model

The shared governance model faces a number of challenges. Certainly one challenge is that of identifying and developing a team of committed people to achieve the desired outcome of a integrated regional health care system. This includes obtaining and maintaining leadership commitment during economic stress, particularly in small institutions. Leaders acknowledge that their work together enhances their ability to thrive as they move toward sharing resources and development programs. Another challenge is that of determining how to support unit-level stakeholders. Although unit-level staff involvement is critical, leaders recognize that unit-level performance alone cannot work: Only a team guided and nurtured by strong leadership can foster changes. A patient- and family-centered delivery system across the region can only be accomplished with the commitment and involvement of everyone affected by the system — experts at the unit level as well as physicians, key community stakeholders, payers, and patients and their families.

Another challenge is that of coping with the stress and tension that change can produce in people at all levels of the organization. (See chapter 7.) Transforming consortium member organizations from conventional hierarchial structures to empowered structures is difficult, and it is critical that the institution plan actions to decrease the stress associated with resistance to change. Education is one means of accomplishing this. Education helps people focus on and clarify what is best practice for patients and their families, rather than on what is best for "me" or "my department." The consortium partners learn that turf issues fall away during interactive processes that support discovery of what each person brings to the change and alignment with the outcome to be achieved. With acceptance of and commitment to change, energy can be directed toward new strategies to solve problems for desired outcomes. Today, work teams are seeing results and outcomes that improve patient and family health. These successes create positive energy that neutralizes negative energy emanating from those who are resistant to change. The key role of leadership in this process is to facilitate, empower (within identified parameters), and publicly recognize positive outcomes that affect patient care through improved quality at efficient cost.

Aadalen discusses how the shared governance structure can help consortium members face their individual challenges and begin to understand and define their role in the partnership:

The shared governance structure and guiding principles of interactive management and systems thinking enhance the member partner's ability to dialogue and learn about their commonalities and unique differences while strategically planning for initiatives related to their vision. Partners gain a sense of appreciation for each other's role in designing an integrated regional health care system across south central Minnesota, and they learn how their relationships and work together result in cost efficiencies, improved quality outcomes, and a work force prepared for future needs. Trust, respect, and appreciation for talents and competencies do not occur without struggle and difficulty. Many traditions based on competition had to be explored, dismantled, and reestablished as collaborative practices and structures evolved. The shared leadership and vision for an improved, integrated regional health care system results in the following learnings and practices:

- Establish a "we" approach and consortiumwide thinking with shared accountability
- Maintain an advocacy relationship among member organizations and educational partners
- Rotate facilitator and leader roles among the member partners for the coordinating council and executive committee
- Develop guidelines for individual committee members to select or replace the chairpersons
- Provide continuous opportunities for personal and team accountability providing ongoing support through the decentralized governance process
- Involve physicians, academic faculty, unit staff, and allied health professionals according to clinical practices and interests as committee members or liaisons to committees
- Develop a formal reporting schedule for committee activity, productivity, and participation by members
- Apply principles of interorganizational structure and shared governance to enhance the probability that consortiumwide goals will be achieved

The shared governance structure strengthens relationships between the partner members and their communities. It provides opportunities for focused, innovative, interdisciplinary consumer inclusive structures, which allow unit-level staff and leaders to achieve interventions for improved patient care services within and between institutions. Organizational productivity is enhanced as a result of collective thinking, and shared learning and accountability. The structure encourages dialogue and strategic thinking which often result in sharing of both human and technological resources. Organizational and community agency leaders express stronger readiness for regional integrated service networks as proposed by health care reform initiatives. Members learn new ways of working together while changing internal structures of each organization to accommodate these learnings and improved services within and across community boundaries. The structure allows them to forge new relationships within the region and liberate indigenous energy, creativity, and leadership.

Shared education programs designed to teach principles of leadership empowerment influence the culture for clinical learning within each member hospital. Academic faculty, managers, clinicians, unit staff, and students together learn concepts of direct communication, relationship management, delegation, problem solving, and negotiating expectations. As a result of the shared learning, baccalaureate and practical nursing faculty now collaborate with nurse managers in planning clinical experiences for students. A goal of their collaborative efforts is innovative clinical assignments to partner baccalaureate and practical nursing students in preparation for practice partnerships when students graduate.

Another unique feature of the partnership is the joint service and education appointment of the consortium director. This appointment is important to strengthening relationships between service and education members as they together design curriculum and practice experiences to meet the current and future clinical work force demands of a regional health care system. The joint appointment gives the director access to the college's strategic planning committee, faculty meetings, and undergraduate curriculum design and course instruction. Convener and facilitator for the LPN-BSN Task Force, member of the steering committee developing the master's in nursing program, and collaborator in the joint development of the graduate Health Policy and Nursing and Family Core sequence have been some of the opportunities resulting from the joint appointment. These activities have evolved over time, in the spirit of joint work force outcomes. Faculty from the academic institutions are members of several hospital clinical committees and often fill a clinician role in order to maintain their practice knowledge and skills.

Outcomes of Health BOND

Productive, effective, and appropriate outcomes give Health BOND the incentive to move ahead proactively rather than reactively. Outcomes for member hospitals include:

• Decreased length of stay and cost for services for specific patient populations

- Established continuum of services for cardiac patients between Abbott-Northwestern Hospital, in Minneapolis, and the consortium hospitals
- Improved utilization of professional and support caregivers
- Increased sharing of human and educational resources
- Decreased reordering of clinical laboratory and X-ray procedures for patients moving between hospitals
- Strengthened physician and trustee relationships and involvement
- Improved caregiver satisfaction, improved communication between hospital leaders and unit-level staff
- Strengthened computer networks between hospitals

Outcomes for educational partners include:

- Improved communication between service and education
- Increased satisfaction for student nurse hospital-based experience
- Established master's of nursing program
- Established service and education joint appointments
- Increased faculty involvement on hospital committees
- Work groups initiated to identify educational needs appropriate for future professional and technical work force

To sustain momentum for these initiatives and realize outcomes for improved community and regional health status, Health BOND leaders must continue to provide support and commitment facilitating collaborative, interorganizational, and intercommunity work teams. The team relationships are necessary to achieve their collective desire to improve access to health services for rural populations in south central Minnesota while maintaining quality and decreasing or stabilizing cost. Although this partnership appears to be well integrated into the fabric of the Health BOND organizations and educational partners, economic forces threaten to erode relationships. This is an ongoing challenge because the relationships remain voluntary. The partnership's future role is oriented toward creating new opportunities for achieving unidentified potentials for the greater good of the institutions and communities within the region by sharing lessons learned from telling their story and by helping teams from other health care organizations and educational institutions to replicate their process and shared governance model.

Being a part of the team process, not only in creating the vision but also in seeing it become reality, is enormously rewarding. Seeing the reality of the vision unfold and recognizing that the process is continuous, leaders of Health BOND are constantly asking: "What needs to be reshaped to continue to achieve shared potentials that benefit the patients and their families, the organizations, the communities, and the region?"

References

1. Ackoff, R. Interactive Planning Model. SHNP education program, Orlando, FL, Sept. 1989.

2. Stamps, P. L., and Piedmont, E. B. *Nurses and Work Satisfaction: An Index for Measurement.* Ann Arbor, MI: Health Administration Press, 1986.

Chapter 13

District of Columbia General Hospital

The District of Columbia General Hospital (DCGH) is located in the nation's capitol, a city plagued by political change and economic strife. The constant state of pandemonium that characterizes DCGH's external environment imposes a great deal of pressure on the hospital's internal operations. As the only acute care public hospital in the city, DCGH is constantly challenged with finding creative ways to care for patients who are without the ability to pay. However, the turbulent external environment in which most DCGH patients and employees live is just one factor influencing the outlook of people inside the hospital. DCGH staff are under constant review from a variety of stakeholders having an impact on hospital operations, including regulators such as the federal agency certifying eligibility to treat Medicare and Medicaid patients. Additionally, overall control of the hospital has changed within the past decade due to internal restructuring, and the decision to place the hospital under the mayor's direct authority has virtually eliminated the control once exercised by the hospital's commission. This chapter looks at the cultural transformation taking place at DCGH and how it is affecting the lives of both staff and patients.

• Achieving Cultural Transformation through Patient-Centered Care

Amidst internal and external turmoil, in the past five years a cultural transformation brought about by implementation of patient-centered care (PCC) is spearheading a change in attitude among employees that will lead DCGH

Chapter 13 was prepared by Chloe Barzey, formerly a consultant with the Center of Applied Research in Philadelphia, who worked with DCGH during PCCDS development and implementation. Presently, she is a consultant with A. T. Kearney, Inc. in Atlanta. A special thank-you is given to Carolyn Hunt, RN, MS, and Gloria Jacks, RN, former PCCDS project staff, for their efforts in facilitating this chapter.

into the next decade. The change to PCC was the result of a grant from the Strengthening Hospital Nursing: Program to Improve Patient Care (supported by The Robert Wood Johnson Foundation and The Pew Charitable Trusts), which started in nursing and then expanded to become hospitalwide.

The transformation process began by first identifying what PCC means to the hospital's staff and patients. Then, using pilot units within the hospital to test PCC concepts, DCGH set a clear definition of what it hoped to accomplish through its PCC program. Many different disciplines collaborated to develop a PCC model that people from all levels of the hospital could accept.

The primary objective of DCGH's Patient-Centered Care Delivery System (PCCDS) is to coordinate care at the unit level, with the patient as the central focus. PCCDS integrates multidisciplinary collaboration and organizational team learning to ensure delivery of high-quality care. As a result of the PCCDS, the hospital has:

- Initiated hospitalwide professional development and recognition efforts
- Involved patients in focus groups to learn about their perceptions and expectations of service
- Achieved decreased length of stay and cost of service for specific patient populations
- Strengthened physician involvement, including residents, at the unit level for patient care improvements
- Strengthened the involvement of the District of Columbia commissioners in improvement of services
- Improved relationships with the schools of nursing and medicine
- Increased caregiver satisfaction and facilitated the caregiver's ability to improve care delivery during times of economic stress, including work force reduction activities

The result is a cultural transformation affecting the work and attitude of people at every organizational level. Evidence of its impact can be found in their own words. Nellie Robinson, former associate administrator of nursing (now assistant executive director for patient care services, Howard University Hospital, also in Washington, DC), describes the greatest challenge in implementing the program:

We thought about what could be a common factor of interest among internal and external stakeholders. It would have to be the patient. We presented core concepts at meetings that were already in place. For example, at medical executive committee meetings, we discussed operational issues with invited representatives from other disciplines present. Our greatest challenge was building trust. In an institution where leadership changes often, it is hard to let people know that you are serious . . . to be effective, we had to walk the talk.

We started by defining patient-centered care and what it meant to each of us; what it meant across services, not just in nursing; what it meant to the hospital; and, ultimately, what it would mean to the patients and their families. The goal was that every facet of hospital care be targeted for improvement from the viewpoint of the patients' concerns.

Anne Murchland, clinical specialist, department of maternal children health, praises the influence of the collaborative care committee:

> I think if there were one thing that I really believe moved us ahead, it was the collaborative care committee . . . it cut through so much bureaucracy and red tape. Staff could say, "This is the problem that we are having from your department in relation on this one item." It is wonderful when someone is there to either explain it, collaborate over it, or take it back to their department and then bring in some type of resolution at the next meeting.

Pamela Copeland, risk manager and acting director for legal risk services, offers this perspective on patient-centeredness:

> As we have moved towards patient-centeredness, there's more of a collaborative effort as it relates to taking care of the patient. What I have noticed especially as a result of being patient focused is that there are less risks to manage. This I attribute to more teamwork by creating a winning situation for the patient and the institution.

Other people at DCGH spoke of the impact of patient-centered care on employee morale. Michael Marby, administrative sergeant, hospital police, explains that for the many employees who had survived years of changes in management and administrative teams, PCC brought an opportunity to participate in the process. "The great thing about the patient-centered care projects [is] that some of these people got an award; they finally were heard." Lawrence Johnson, medical director, adds:

> People saw themselves as being part of something that was of value to the institution; something that ultimately would achieve the kinds of results that they wanted. . . . What we did was not so much innovation but rediscovery — getting back to basics to reconfirm what had initially attracted many of us to the healing profession to begin with: concern for others, inquisitiveness, and a scientific approach to problem solving.

• Sharing the Lessons Learned

The cultural transformation at DCGH is an ongoing process. As people continue to learn to collaborate in a dynamic environment, they are faced with new challenges for which they need innovative solutions. DCGH staff have learned many valuable lessons that staffs in other organizations undergoing change will find useful. One of these lessons is that there is no value to be gained in introducing the organization's mission or vision until time has been taken to assess where each individual feels he or she belongs in the organization. Other lessons include:

- Providing frequent, redundant information through weekly communication strategies such as internal newsletters, increased access to managers and executive leaders, and routine employee forms for information and conversation
- Implementing an education program for all levels of staff in all departments in order to promote the understanding of a PCC environment paying particular attention to caregivers and support staff at the unit level
- Providing opportunities for emotional honesty by being sensitive to the resources that caregivers need as they learn to work with interdisciplinary groups
- Designing a reward and recognition program that shows appreciation to all caregivers (nurses, physicians, and other professionals) and support staff who contribute to improving patient care

As Rachel Smith, former director for nursing education and cochair of the Patient-Centered Hospital Environment Committee, puts it "Employees must be valued and recognized for their contributions on a regular basis." Staff managers who are a part of PCCD agree, it is important to say thank you several times a day. When a hospital is experiencing economic stress, like DCGH, a thank you can be as important as a material reward.

Howard Jessamy, chair of the Advisory Committee for the Patient-Centered Care Delivery System, District of Columbia Hospital Association, adds that the PCC process can motivate employees:

Patient-centered care is by no means a panacea for all of the ills at DCGH, but it is an important component for improving our patient care. It is a means of bringing a more motivated employee into the mission and the vision by more than just a paycheck.

Hank Primas, associate director, environmental services, stresses the importance of personal recognition:

Housekeepers are professionals; they take pride in their work and their job. Here, we tell them thank-you and try to treat them as people, rather than as a stereotype which people figure housekeepers ought to be. I stay motivated; I want this to be one of the best-looking hospitals around.

Mark Chastang, former executive director (now president/CEO, East Orange General Hospital), underscores the notion that every employee needs to be invited to become part of the organization's vision:

> It is very important to create dreams that others will willingly adopt. Effective leadership helps the organization fashion a vision or a dream and persuade people to adopt it — or to dream for themselves — and assist them in achieving it.
>
> People can be very satisfied on a battlefield — a MASH unit, for example. People can be extremely motivated about giving patient care in the most difficult circumstances that you can imagine. DC General is a battlefield. Inspired people can achieve anything.

• Looking Ahead

Looking ahead to the year 2010, DCGH staff members discuss what should happen in the coming years to make DCGH a hospital of choice and a model for patient-centered care throughout the nation.

Smith identified a range of changes she would like to see the organization make in the next few years:

> The organization was restructured to make salaries of employees and shareholders tied to performance; the board of directors became comprised of at least 50 percent community representatives; [the] organization committed to at least 50 percent succession management; the organization moved to cross-train employees and had [a] well-defined employee development plan; and the organization adopted [a] shared governance model and eliminated multiple layers of management.

Primas would like to see hospital management patterned after private industry:

> . . . ideas and innovations are rewarded, not only in technology but also in dealing with people. For example, "Here's your performance appraisal, you fill it out, tell me what it should be."

Barbara Hunt, nurse manager for pediatric emergency room and pediatric outpatient department, looks forward to an improved information system and greater community outreach and involvement:

> We changed the computer system so that information is updated and it takes registration two minutes to register (currently it could take hours for patients with extenuating circumstances). We did more to reach out

to the public. We had a van that would go out to a church and give immunizations. DC General has grandmother volunteers; we have a lot of latchkey kids and our grandmothers are there. A hot line lets those kids call grandmom if they get scared before mom showed up. The teenagers in the community are working in this role also.

Copeland sees a true team approach to patient care and hospital involvement with the community as key elements of the hospital's future role:

> There are no walls as it relates to the departmental divides that exist . . . the wall between physicians and nurses has really eroded and we have a truly team approach to the patient (with everyone recognized by their area of expertise). We see a lot more in terms of the outpatient area being celebrated. The institution is more involved with the community and solicits the community more than in the past. We have shown the country that, while individuals may have the unfortunate status of being uninsured, they can produce a lot in terms of being healthy citizens in this country, and they are worth saving and investing in. The role of the hospital is being a social agent as opposed to being the reactor to a social situation.

Marby looks to a future where communication between administration and staff is open and personal:

> There are monthly meetings in each division where the executive staff listen to the views of the employee, what they think needs to be improved and to relieve them of fears that they may have in reference to their jobs. There is an open-door policy.

Shirley Edwards, acting associate administrator of nursing, focuses on the role of patient education:

> We have educated the patient concerning a healthier lifestyle and prevention of disease, so that they are a partner in their own self-care.

Richard Lopez, director of substance abuse program, hopes for a leadership that will care for its staff:

> The hospital has compassion, technical expertise, a good financial base, and can provide effective services without compromising quality patient care. Its leadership is made of creative problem solvers, [who] are flexible, support their staff, and provide them with the things that they need. Caring for the staff is translated to caring for the patient.

And finally, Chastang, perhaps mindful of DCGH's unique position within its troubled community, sees the need to define patient-centered care according to the needs of the specific population it serves:

> The future is not one of growth and expansion; the future is one that is premised on limited resources. Patient-centeredness will have to be redefined around compelling community interests, such as care and treatment of AIDS victims, prisoners, drug abusers, and other major social problems. So patient-centeredness is going to have two compelling issues driving it for the future: one is limited resources, and the other is social problems that are overwhelming the government and the community.

Chapter 14

Vanderbilt University Medical Center

Leadership and staff at the Vanderbilt University Medical Center (VUMC) together created the Center for Patient Care Innovation (CPCI) to facilitate team decision making in operational and clinical management issues. This chapter describes CPCI and the accomplishments it supports, and discusses what the Vanderbilt leadership and participants learned from this innovation.

• Center for Patient Care Innovation

CPCI is dedicated to dreams, imagination, and visions as primary tools for innovation and improvement. Initiated as part of Vanderbilt University Hospital's SHNP project, CPCI was conceived by leadership, physicians, clinical nurses, nurse educators, and nurse researchers interested in:

- Improving delivery of patient care
- Producing better solutions to systems problems
- Fostering a satisfying work environment for all care providers

Through its dedicated staff, CPCI advises, facilitates, coaches, and evaluates clinical projects and innovations for systems improvement throughout VUMC. Three objectives guide CPCI:

1. To promote innovation and creativity at all levels of Vanderbilt University Hospital and The Vanderbilt Clinic
2. To facilitate continuous improvement in the operational and clinical management of patient care services

Special appreciation is given to Wendy L. Baker, former director of CPCI and staff associate, Office of the Senior Director, University of Michigan Hospital, Ann Arbor, who interviewed contributors to this chapter and reported their comments.

3. To further vertical and horizontal integration of the hospital and clinic patient care delivery systems guided by the principles of patient-focused care (PFC) and teachings from facilitative leadership (FL).

PFC and FL are key elements of CPCI. PFC principles include the restructure of service delivery for a specific patient population using a decentralized approach; redesign of jobs and work processes to meet the needs of that population; creation of shared work for multiskilled staff; elimination of non-value-added activities in hospitals to support a more responsive service delivery system; and establishment of parameters, criteria, or indicators for monitoring results. Developed by Interaction Associates, Inc., San Francisco, and modified by CPCI, FL is a course emphasizing collaborative planning and meeting skills and techniques. It enables managers and project leaders to practice facilitation skills and receive feedback on their abilities. The course provides participants an opportunity to understand the connection between their work at the unit or department level and the clinical outcomes for patients.

• Accomplishments Supported by CPCI

The CPCI supports a variety of accomplishments. These include:

- The redesign and restructure of inpatient units and central departments, focusing on PFC. PFC involves decentralizing specific patient units of the hospital so that services are brought to the patient rather than bringing the patient to the services. It is a patient needs-driven model of care promoting cost efficiencies and service quality.[1]
- The restructure of staff and manager roles strengthening PFC and collaborative care. Role design and redesign are determined for both professional and support staff by the needs of the patient.
- Realization of a collaborative care and case management model for delivery of patient services, including collaborative pathways (a version of clinical pathways).
- Implementation of a consultation service throughout VUMC in areas such as project management, group process, meeting planning, teamwork, and work and role redesign.
- Creation of a comprehensive team and leadership development program (facilitative leadership).
- Implementation of an interdisciplinary shared governance model that provides opportunities to move decision making closer to the level of the people doing the work.
- Design of a computerized documentation system — Pathways™ — that decreases nurse charting time and links the use of collaborative pathways to continuous quality improvement (CQI) efforts.[2]

- Initiation of an evaluation program that focuses on the impact of these and other initiatives on cost, quality, and patient satisfaction.

• Insights of Executive Leadership

Norman Urmy, executive director; Judy Spinella, director/COO; and Stephen Entman, professor/vice-chair, obstetrics and gynecology, were change agents in the process at VUMC. In this section, they discuss some of the motivational forces that influenced them to refine their vision, change their management style, and involve physicians early in the change process. They also offer thoughts on the skills and values of transformational leaders.

Refining the Vision

Urmy describes the history of his vision for a patient needs-responsive system and the impact on his thinking of the Patient-Focused Care Consortium (PFCC), led by J. Philip Lathrop:

> My vision for a patient needs-responsive system of care dates back to 1974 while I was working in New York. At that time, I developed ideas about the integration of medical, nursing, and administrative leadership. Pressured by an environment of financial stress, we [hospital leadership] knew we had to change and the organization had too many bureaucratic layers. The motivation in 1974 was purely financially driven. The motivation in the 1990s continues to be financial but with attention to patient needs. Learning about [the] Patient Focused Care Consortium (PFCC), led by J. Philip Lathrop, vice-president for Booz Allen Consultants, recalled my thinking of 1974. I wanted to be part of the group of hospitals implementing those principles and setting new directions for delivering patient care services. Being a member of the consortium meant changing the objectives for the VUMC from centralized services to more decentralized approaches. We accepted things would change in a radical way, since PFC does away with traditional thinking and places the focus on patient needs rather than on the department or discipline.
>
> The description of a hospital by J. Philip Lathrop and dialogue with members of the PFCC provided new insights and guidance for change at the medical center. For example, he described the number of job tasks and steps to get an X ray. It [the PFC description] fit with what I've heard for many years and fit with what I knew intuitively as an efficient way of working. Flowcharting the steps involved in an X-ray procedure, one realizes that 63 to 70 percent of work has to do with things that are not related to taking an X ray. Understanding the need

to create efficiencies, we decided to decentralize and implement the PFC concept, starting with orthopedic services. We had some advantages including space, dollars, time, and talented people to make the change. Thinking back, it would have been difficult to accomplish the orthopedics redesign if we didn't have the dollars and people to invest. [The orthopedic unit is designed with many of the patient support services directly on the unit, such as admission and discharge functions, routine laboratory, and X-ray facilities. The philosophy supports meeting the services of the patient on the unit by a consistent team of care providers in a cost-efficient manner.]

Urmy acknowledges that the advent of Tennessee's managed care (Tenn Care) and potential capitated payment system for some patients is increasing financial concerns for VUMC because of the heavy emphasis on reducing utilization of services with the potential to drastically reduce revenues. He says: "PFC will enhance our ability to strategically plan how to respond to these pressures. Implementing the PFC, the hospital has designed shared work roles by training support staff with multiple skills." For example, some unit managers and unit clerks share roles and job functions. Multiskilled patient service support staff are paired with a professional nurse to meet the needs of a group of patients. These clinical partnerships have resulted in a change in staff skill mix on a particular inpatient unit, reducing salary costs and sometimes full-time equivalent staff positions. This means a cost decrease for patient services to that patient population. Cost reductions are demonstrated through organizational performance reports developed by information services staff. Along with the restructuring activities, the partnerships have implemented many CQI strategies to create further cost efficiencies while maintaining a high standard of quality. Nurses, physicians, and other disciplines have been involved directly and intimately in deciding these changes, including development of new roles and service delivery methods.

Spinella further explains how PFCC principles helped VUMC leadership formulate a new way of thinking about patient care service delivery:

PFCC helped us define our vision and direction initially for orthopedic services and now throughout the medical center. SHNP helped us with things we wanted to promulgate in the organization such as FL and unit boards. [Unit boards bring together unit staff, managers, and administrators to address clinical and operational issues. Many of them are interdisciplinary and interdepartmental, and are based on Ackoff's concept of the circular organization.[3]] Resources such as dedicated staff, materials, and consultants for innovation and improvement were supported by the CPCI.

Urmy and Spinella agree on the value of having been part of the PFCC:

We had an opportunity over a year time frame to discuss a "straw man" PFC model with the consortium group. This process gave us ideas for direction in initiating the project at Vanderbilt. It also provided us time to identify the resources, both human and other, we would need to achieve a desirable end product.

Entman adds that "PFC and CPCI provided opportunities for financial staff and patient care staff to identify mutual goals and to work together in different ways." One example of this collaboration is the multidisciplinary obstetrical management team (MOM). Administrators, nurses, and physicians jointly designed the team, and financial and information systems staff designed the quality and cost-monitoring and reporting mechanisms. Composed of seven physicians and four RN care coordinators (case managers), MOM manages the prenatal care of approximately 400 clinic patients, slightly less than 50 percent of the maternity patient population at the medical center.[4] The care coordinators, teamed with certain physicians, are responsible for the majority of the hands-on prenatal care and case management; an attending physician provides hands-on care for high-risk patients. The model promotes a partnership between physicians and nurses as they pursue the same goal. Patients receive more individualized attention, increased educational episodes for preparing for their new baby, and enhanced quality of care outcomes. The result is that the hospital and clinic are realizing cost efficiencies, and the care providers are finding increased satisfaction with their contribution to improved outcomes for prenatal patients.

Adjusting Managerial Style

The management philosophy embraced by the Vanderbilt leadership team is a part of the FL course. It stresses collaboration and team decision making, bringing together the people closest to problems — the "real experts" — to design solutions. The philosophy is role-modeled by the VUMC leadership team as they provide managers and project leaders in-house education to help them contribute successfully to strategic unit- and department-level decisions.

Urmy describes how his management style and role have changed:

Seeing the need to decentralize decision-making processes to fit with the principles of PFC, I somehow had to become a check point in the process of management, rather than an approval body, although there are times when I am required to be the approval body. Again, my desire in 1974 to create a plan for a "minihospital" with nursing–hospital administrator teams became the basis for my thinking and the model for designing a different management system and adapting my leadership style. Like many administrators, my style typically has been to be directive; I now find myself using more facilitating, mentoring, and supporting skills along with directive skills.

Spinella's initial position was executive director for nursing services, which included traditional department of nursing responsibilities. Envisioning a broader management model, her role and responsibilities expanded to include patient care services and then to incorporate the role of chief operating officer. Her role change was particularly meaningful in the development of the interdisciplinary shared governance in patient care services and the collaborative patient care delivery model. She explains:

I thought if I do PFC right, I might get rid of the [my] job. Rather than getting rid of the job, the job functions actually expanded. My role changed to managing interactions, relationships, and functions across departments instead of managing specific people and operational details—the job will be needed for a long time.

Involving Physicians

Physician involvement in the health care organization's change process is essential to its success. Entman discusses the need to define the medical leader's role in the change process and the challenges inherent in soliciting physician involvement:

The Russell Ackoff lecture[5] was one of the most illuminating points of my life; it wasn't what he said, but more what I saw. It was the first time I'd heard anyone talk about how and why people think differently. Rather than a demand for transformation, the need was to identify the role of the medical leader . . . he moved from the nebulous to defined roles. We still need aspects of the traditional role; although it is often adversarial, it establishes boundaries. If you don't have definition you can't transform. It's also important to have defined goals—a vision.

The need for medical leadership to take time to think and be contemplative is important to a change initiative that is of the magnitude occurring at Vanderbilt. For example, Allen Kaiser, who has a clinical leadership position reporting directly to the chief of medicine, was given time specifically to think out issues and identify improvements in medical services.

The relationship of physicians to the hospital in an academic setting presents a difficulty in promoting and sustaining change. The VUH and Vanderbilt Clinic staff are the executive director's employees. Asking a physician to get involved requires a significant investment on his or her part. As responsibilities increase, physicians want to be able to use their time more efficiently. Many want to achieve better balance in their life between work, family, and recreation. I am hopeful that working more efficiently as an organization, this balance will be more attainable. The failure to involve MDs in formulating the mission and vision, and failure to acknowledge that the VUMC faculty have conflicting roles that are mutually exclusive, has been a problem. That tension is played out like this: During the time the faculty member is functioning as a clinician, the highest goal is patient care. But the "lab rats," colleagues more interested in research, laugh at that; it's the attitude that is conveyed to staff that's a problem. The key is acknowledgement of diverse roles of faculty. During the time when you're doing patient care, that care has to come first, but traditionally the mission of the VUM has focused emphasis on research. Now, the VUH [Vanderbilt University Hospital] and The Vanderbilt Clinic focus is clinical practice. The two goals are becoming more synergistic.

Spinella focuses on the effort at VUH to involve physicians in the transformation:

We clearly recognized that leadership for innovation requires an investment of money and time for everyone, including the medical staff. Recognizing the importance of their involvement early in the process, the VUH leadership has made a significant effort to understand how to involve physicians by identifying the positive effects for their patients. Initially, they captured the attention of a "chosen few." Once they were able to demonstrate positive quality and cost outcomes, particularly with their collaborative care and case management model, they were able to enlist many others. Although they have many successes with physician involvement, this continues to be a struggle, particularly with the complexity of residents and medical students.

Urmy underscores the need for physician involvement early on:

There was a feeling of dis-empowerment by the physicians while management was getting its act together. They [physicians] were not initially built into the structure. If I had to do it over, I'd have more members of the medical staff at [the] table with us developing the mission and vision, including the FL course. A structure is needed that defines the role of the physician and allows them to feel the empowerment they need to carry out those roles.

Assessing the Skills and Values of Transformational Leaders

Having been change agents, Urmy, Spinella, and Entman have much to say about the skills needed to be a transformational leader.

Urmy emphasizes the willingness to communicate and the ability to work with others:

> The "great" management theory is the leader controls the development of ideas and that authoritarian management does not work because it does not invite feedback. Transformational leaders have to be skilled listeners, and value and solicit feedback. Listening means being able to plug in so that you're not just driving your own personal vision. The leader should be able to describe the vision, present ideas, and challenge people in a positive way. The leader must value innovation, believe that change is good and necessary, and value the ideas of other people.
>
> As a leader I have found that jargon is not conducive to direction or effective management. The focus on jargon taps into the struggle for definition. It is my opinion that using jargon gives a sense that there is no one leading.

Entman stresses the importance of clarity of vision:

> Clarity of vision is an important skill of transformational leaders. They should provide definition of roles for others and boundaries within which others can operate more independently. Leaders must be clear when their role is advisory and when they must be the decision maker. Most difficulties we experienced during this change process resulted from people not being fully prepared for the new team decision-making role. The root cause, I believe, was that people didn't know what their role was or who was making decisions.
>
> I agree . . . that jargon is not helpful. Words carry a lot. Physicians often feel assaulted during change processes that they do not understand and jargon just exacerbates the problem. Most physicians and staff feel the new titles and words used are meant to keep them from understanding. For example, the new title manager, patient care services. What does it mean? It is more important that we work out the functions of the role and communicate those functions. Roles should be designed around the work or service to the patient rather than the role driving the work.

Spinella focuses on the necessity of holding people accountable for translating vision into outcomes:

> Leaders need to learn how to hold people accountable, particularly in a collaborative, interdisciplinary model. They must prepare them for

accountability and provide them opportunities to learn the knowledge and skills they need and the experiences to be accountable. Some people will agree with and enjoy accountability; others will just go along or possibly resist it. If the leader doesn't hold people accountable for how the vision translates into outcomes, nothing will change. Top-down and bottom-up input and endorsement is needed to change how accountability is viewed for everyone to be accountable, not only the executive staff. Defining outcomes and objectives is a skill key to getting people involved and facilitating their understanding of how they make a difference.

• Learnings from the Change Process at VUMC

Learnings are a source of reflection and re-vision that can be shared with others to facilitate development without experiencing some of the disappointments of change. The learnings presented below are based on an aggregation of responses from the Vanderbilt participants.

- Involve people at all levels of the organization, particularly those who will be affected by change.
- Integrate the academic, educational, and research missions into one mission.
- Take time to agree on how to work together to achieve a desired end.
- Develop a mechanism to communicate the vision so that others can understand and endorse it, and do not assume that everyone will agree with it.
- Ask "What did we learn?" at numerous intervals throughout the change process.
- Recognize that some issues can be eliminated by asking questions differently. For example: "As we move forward with this change, how can you help us?"
- Talk about mistakes and understand why they happened.
- Offer simple and clear answers, even if questions are complex.
- Establish common terminology that can be understood by clinicians and operational people, and refrain from using jargon.
- Strengthen listening skills by listening for what is *not* said.
- Design information systems to collect clinical and operational data early in the process. Data are essential in comparing "what was" with "what is" and for showing effective progress and constant improvement.

VUMC's collaborative, interdisciplinary restructuring efforts are resulting in patient care services that are constantly improving and costs that are decreasing while quality is being maintained at a high standard. These desired outcomes have expanded the new patient care delivery model based on the principles of PFC and work and role redesign to 26 care units and 6 central departments.[6] Each area has:

- Defined clinical care processes and outcomes along with managed care standards
- Delegated tasks to the least expensive care provider most trained in the principles of PFC
- Decentralized staff and management of the most frequently used ancillary support and administrative functions
- Reduced organizational layers and broadened the span of control to streamline decision making
- Reduced and eliminated process complexities through process redesign and technology applications

A collaborative organizational design process using an interdisciplinary team of clinical staff and administrators is revisioning the potential to create a more efficient PFC system that values patients and other customers. It is creating a Center for Continuous Learning and Improvement which seeks opportunities for new quality initiatives, develops performance-based compensation and evaluation for all levels of staff, implements computer-based patient records from access to care through discharge from care, and standardizes product supply and selection.[7] The VUMC has embraced innovative opportunities by changing perceptions of risk and consequences. It has learned what it means to change and has found a balance between tradition and transformation.

References

1. Moore, N., and Komras, H. *Patient-Focused Healing: Integrating Caring and Curing in Health Care.* San Francisco: Jossey-Bass, 1993.

2. Vanderbilt University Medical Center: looks to collaborative care to manage patient care. *Strengthening* 1(3):5, 7, Winter 1994.

3. Ackoff, R. L. *Creating the Corporate Future.* New York City: John Wiley and Sons, 1981.

4. Vanderbilt University Medical Center: looks to collaborative care to manage patient care.

5. Ackoff, R. Interactive Planning Model. SHNP education program, Orlando, FL, Sept. 1989.

6. Vanderbilt University Medical Center: looks to collaborative care to manage patient care.

7. National Program Office. *Strengthening Hospital Nursing: A Program to Improve Patient Care National Meeting Brochure and Meeting Resource Notebook.* St. Petersburg, FL: The Robert Wood Johnson Foundation and The Pew Charitable Trusts, Fall 1994.

Chapter 15

Northeast Health Consortium

The Northeast Health Consortium, in Rockport, Maine, is a small community health care system that comprises acute care, long-term care, and home care facilities. With approximately 1,000 employees, it is the largest employer in Knox County. Historically, the community of Rockport has attracted many visionary thinkers, several of whom have focused on health and social welfare. This chapter describes Northeast Health Consortium's struggle to design an integrated care system.

• An Integrated Care System for Community Health

Since the announcement of the Strengthening Hospital Nursing Program (SHNP) in 1989, health care system leadership in Rockport has spent many hours developing the Northeast Health Consortium for Integrated Care. The consortium is composed of Camden Health Care Center, in Camden; Kno-Wal-Lin Home Care and The Knox Center for Long Term Care, a department of Penobscot Bay Medical Center, both in Rockland; and Penobscot Bay Medical Center, in Rockport. The goal of the consortium's integrated care project is to coordinate the most efficient use of resources across the entire system in order to deliver appropriate, high-quality, and affordable health care to the people of the region. Consortium members work together through:

- An integrated information system
- Case coordination for specific patient populations with member facilities, payers, and other providers

Chapter 15 was prepared by Paula Delahanty, RN, director, quality management department, Penobscot Bay Medical Center, Rockport, Maine, and former project director, Integrated Care System, Northeast Health Consortium, Rockport, Maine. Judith Coffin, administrative assistant, Penobscot Bay Medical Center, Rockport, Maine, is acknowledged for her valuable review and editing.

- An integrated transfer process utilizing care pathways, systemwide refer-
  rals, and universal discharge and transfer procedures
- Integrated education utilizing education personnel networks, shared education resources, and systemwide program development

The consortium participated in the SHNP from 1989 to 1994.

• Northeast Health Consortium Leadership on the Change Process

Some of the key players in Northeast Health Consortium's efforts to effect
its change process describe below the commitment–resistance tug-of-war that
has characterized the consortium's change effort. Alan Kinne, administrator of Knox Center for Long-Term Care, a division of Penobscot Bay Medical Center, and member of the steering committee for the integrated care
project uses a nautical analogy:

> I have likened our recent venture into the world of health care revitali-
> zation (via the sea of commitment and perseverance) to an ocean cruise.
> Our ship went from the Sea of Tranquility to the Monsoons of Osaka.
> As the administrator of one of our long-term care components, I was
> fortunate to have been a member of the original steering committee.
> During our planning phase, we brought on board those people we felt
> helped to initiate our new course. As we progressed through ad hoc com-
> mittees, we gathered interested and committed people like a rolling snow-
> ball. By the time we submitted our plan and direction for the future,
> we had an enthusiastic group ready for the leadership to move us ahead.
> We then noticed the sky clouding up and the winds and rains threatening.
>   We did not seem to have a single focus from those who were to
> carry us onward. We submitted our plan, received support and
> encouragement nationally, and were told to go forward. I think the real-
> ity of having to implement what we said "set in." We found that those
> claiming to be in agreement and supportive were not ready to make
> the total commitment. We then seemed to drift aimlessly, as our ship
> had no rudder and was floundering amongst the crests and troughs of
> our turbulent sea. We sought professional help to bring us back together
> as a team—the staff, volunteers, trustees, and physicians. This "team"
> was again ready to raise the sails and move ahead, but it appeared that
> the rest of the "crew" did not feel a part of this and began to resist.
> During this period, we made a conscious effort to bring all the new
> trustees and staff up to speed. We wanted to show them the necessity
> of a continued effort to bring our system together as one, in the best
> interest of all those we serve. We had support within each of the "sister

organizations"—the hospital, the long-term care facilities, and the home health agency—but we still did not have the unified commitment of the parent corporation.

Although we were aware of the possibility of mutiny and piracy on our seaward journey, we continued to educate, encourage, and bring together both the people and the corporations that made up our system. Piece by piece, our leadership changed. Along with that came cooperation, acceptance, and commitment to the system as the only way we would be able to meet what is ahead. It is nice to suggest that paradigm shifts, focused direction, critical mass, CQI [continuous quality improvement], TQM [total quality management], and all the other jargon that has surfaced and become the industry buzzwords is what brought us all together. I sincerely do not believe there is any one single item or process that brought us through the troubled waters and into calmer seas. It is my feeling we all came to understand [that] to survive and prepare ourselves to meet the coming changes in the practice of medicine and the delivery of health care, we must coalesce. We also realized that once we were all together the only thing left was to go ahead and "do it."

For our health system, this project has served as a major organizational turning point. To even agree on a vision, an entire cultural change was required. As we were deep in the midst of cultural change, major leadership roles were vacated. These vacant roles caused or intensified frustration, but also created opportunities.

Joanne Smith, facilitator and case coordinator for the medical, surgical, and orthopedic unit of Penobscot Bay Medical Center, describes her roller coaster experience with cultural practice patterns and leadership changes:

I joined the integrated care project staff in March of 1993 as orthopedic facilitator mainly because the staff had changed and the new project director was a person I had worked with previously and for whom I had tremendous respect. During this time, the acute care aspect of our organization was experiencing a leadership vacuum (both chief executive officer [CEO] and the vice-president of nursing were being recruited) and our proposal for integrated care was being redrafted. Included in the new proposal was a refocus on orthopedic care: geographically clustering these patients in one area; recruiting a self-selected staff from in-house; and designing an education plan that broadened the acute care nurse's view of the totality of orthopedic care. Included were "shadow" experiences at physician's offices, physical therapy, operating room postanesthesia care, home health, skilled nursing care, and long-term care.

In this climate, the idea of establishing an orthopedic unit rolled around gathering rumors and resentment. Staff were shown videos about paradigm shifts. Attempts to relate those ideas to staff-level functioning by the project geriatric nurse clinician (who had no rapport with staff or knowledge of their level of functioning) met with confusion. Allowing the staff of the two units currently caring for orthopedic patients to decide among themselves where to locate the new 10-bed orthopedic unit resulted in an impasse. Finally, focus was brought to the problem. All the stakeholders were brought together. A mutually agreed-upon list of priorities was set up and a plan for interviewing and selecting staff was made. (There was a minor procedural battle initially between those who wanted to address delivery of care and staff mix first versus those who wanted to get the unit under way. This was resolved in favor of getting the unit under way.) The speed and enthusiasm with which the staff undertook and accomplished the tasks necessary to operationalize the unit strengthens the supposition that leadership and communication had been the missing pieces.

The establishment of this unit reflects, in many ways, the transformation of the entire organizational culture. A paternalistic, top-down management style presiding over very territorial inner-focused departments is evolving into the communicative and collaborative style that characterizes the orthopedic unit today.

The evolution, encouraged and supported by the consortium's integrated care project and now being driven by the health care climate, has been neither smooth nor painless. Communication at all levels has always been a major problem at our 104-bed acute care facility. This problem possibly stems from times past when unshared information represented power. This attitude, coupled with the lack of a clearly articulated, universally "bought-into" statement of organizational mission and values tended to sabotage any changes regardless of how laudable.

Communication and collaboration continue to affect each other synergistically among patients and caregivers on the unit. Unit-based respiratory therapy and social work further focus care as does use of care pathways, a tool continuing to be revised as orthopedic length of stay [LOS] and other factors change. Staff have begun to communicate with providers outside acute care to coordinate ongoing care; they willingly entertain the possibility of providing education and care for their patients in other settings.

The unit coordinator for the 20-bed unit of which 10 beds are the orthopedic unit provides excellent leadership for change on the unit as well as in the hospital at large. Establishment of the orthopedic unit from the original 20 beds, and the self-selecting staffing, has the unforeseen outcome of some of the remaining staff feeling like "poor relations" of the orthopedic staff. The unit coordinator continues to work to resolve this conflict, utilizing the skills of a consultant to work with the staff.

This 10-bed orthopedic unit is nearing its first anniversary of a very successful beginning. The care is patient focused, interdisciplinary, and collaborative, with a staff that is flexible, willing, and able to role-model. My role continues to be that of a staff member and facilitator working closely with the unit coordinator to address issues that bridge acute care through the orthopedic resource group and the quality management department of the hospital. Currently, we are working together with the quality management department on a project with Blue Cross and Blue Shield of Maine to collect and analyze data on elective joint surgery to bring to our unit the cost/LOS data the nurses traditionally have not considered. Although our relationship has always been smooth, my relationship with other management personnel has not. Now that our CEO and vice-president of nursing are in place, I think that we will see a much finer focus on mission and values. It will not be an easy transition with so many people in the organization at different places in this evolutionary process.

Bill Zuber, director, occupational therapy and physical therapy department of Penobscot Bay Medical Center (and former facilitator for the stroke resource group of the integrated care project) describes his transformational experience as follows:

Participating in this process from the development of the integrated care proposal in late 1990 to the present, I have had the opportunity to see what the many faces and aspects that this process of change brought to a small rural health care organization trying to assemble a vertically integrated continuum of care. At least, I can call it that now. At the time of the initiation of the project, it seemed to me we were just trying to bring everything together to work more smoothly. Having a background as an occupational therapist and a training program that was heavily based in a holistic approach that spanned acute care, rehabilitation, and home care, it all seemed pretty simple to me.

I already worked in all the areas that the project was trying to bring together. I had experienced the frustration of the patient being discharged from acute care and arriving at the rehabilitation center within the same system as a totally new patient that brought no previous history with them. However, I was using the discharge summary I had written at the hospital as my initial evaluation on the rehabilitation unit. Not much usually changed during the 10-minute ambulance ride. And on the occasion that I could also see this patient in their home environment after their rehab stay and encourage them through their initial discouragement upon arriving home and finding that everything was not going to be normal again, and by reminding them of what their function was like while I was treating them at the hospital directly after their stroke, again was a tremendous exception to the norm.

I was soon to learn that my flexibility and vision of an integrated system of "seamless" care system that put at its center the needs of the patient who remained constant as he or she passed through different episodes and levels of care was not the norm for the rest of the fragmented system. I also learned that this is what others across the board envisioned for the system: a seamless, vertically integrated continuum of care.

Serving as a steering committee member (the governing body for the project represented by executive leadership from the member facilities, trustee and physician representatives, and project staff), a member of most of the task forces involved in the work, and historian to the many twists and turns of the project, I had the opportunity to observe many of the challenges, failures, and successes (I would now call both "opportunities for improvement") that this project presented our institution and system. I do distinctly remember turning to a fellow staff person in the education department on the day of the announcement of the award of the SHNP grant in October 1990 and both of us agreeing that the majority of people in the institution really did not have a clue as to what we were committing ourselves to doing, if we were to be truly successful in meeting the original objects that had been set forth.

If I were to sum up the salient points of what I learned about change in going through this project, they would center around the following areas:

- Knowing your personal strengths and weaknesses in communicating effectively.
- Learning how to walk and navigate on ground that is always moving.
- Learning how to press forward to a goal or outcome, even though you do not have a clear definition of what that outcome will be.
- Knowing that by the time you reach the outcome, it will be different from what was initially envisioned.
- Knowing that a process such as this will never be complete, it will continue to evolve. Therefore, you must constantly be reevaluating your objectives to continue to move in the desired direction.

Paula Delahanty, director, quality management department, Penobscot Bay Medical Center (and former project director of the Northeast Consortium for Integrated Care System) summarizes the experience:

This transformational experience has validated the Consortium's original vision of creating a seamless delivery system of patient care across the Consortium institutions. As we are finding, this system is providing strengthened continuity of care for patients, reduced cost of services, and increased satisfaction for care providers, patients, and their families. In order to move toward an integrated system, we found that we needed to work together, putting aside our differences for the interest of the patient and community. When a group of providers position themselves for such a fundamental change (working collaboratively rather than competitively), it is important that leaders of the organizations have a common vision and understand the strategies to transform the environment to one of helping each other for a common purpose. This has not been an easy process for us, however, we are committed and eager to demonstrate that we can change for the benefit of the people we serve.

Part Six

Appendixes

Appendix A

Strengthening Hospital Nursing: A Program to Improve Patient Care

Strengthening Hospital Nursing: A Program to Improve Patient Care (SHNP), jointly sponsored by The Robert Wood Johnson Foundation and The Pew Charitable Trusts, demonstrates that, through the efforts of care providers working together, institutionwide restructuring can facilitate development of innovative models for efficiently and conveniently meeting the needs of patients and their families. In so doing, the program:

- Shows how commitment to new and improved collaborative and interdependent relationships can lead to cocreation — people working together for the purpose of achieving the common desired outcome of improved community health status
- Teaches appropriate use of resources, both human and technological; demonstrates performance efficiencies and patient care efficacy; and champions continuing value and quality improvement
- Emphasizes solidarity among disciplines (for example, nurses, physicians, support staff, and other professionals) from all levels of the organization
- Focuses on new ways to get things done by building a shared vision of what health care systems may be
- Encourages processes of interactive planning, systems thinking, value management, and learning organizations for creating a responsive, adaptable, synergistic, and holistic patient care delivery system
- Describes the effectiveness of a patient-centered philosophy of care and illustrates the value of continuums of care across all care settings — for example, hospital-based, home, long-term, wellness, preventive, and community-based care

---

The views expressed in this overview of the national program are solely those of the authors. Official endorsement by the Robert Wood Johnson Foundation or the Pew Charitable Trusts is not intended and should not be inferred.

• Program Evolution

In the 1980s, changes in health care reimbursement, advances in biomedical technology, and alterations in the profile of hospitalized patients caused an imbalance in the supply of key health professionals and the demands for their service. The Robert Wood Johnson Foundation and The Pew Charitable Trusts wanted to improve cost-effective patient care outcomes by strengthening usage of professional resources, specifically nursing. These foundations hypothesized that institutionwide restructuring might make it possible to address problems that discourage nurses and other professionals from providing cost-effective, optimal patient care services.

In October 1988, the foundations sponsoring SHNP mailed a brochure (Call for Proposal), which outlined the details of the grant application, to nonprofit general hospitals in the United States that called for strengthening hospital nursing for the improvement of patient care. The Call for Proposal announced a two phase grant program for a total of 26.8 million dollars. Phase I would award up to $50,000 to 80 grantees meeting the selection criteria, and Phase II would award up to $1,000,000 to 20 grantees who demonstrated innovative restructuring projects for the improvement of patient care. One million of the 26.8 million dollars was used for the education programs sponsored by SHNP and the remaining funds were used for administrative and technical assistance provided by the national program office in St. Petersburg, Florida.

Hospitals with 300 or more beds were eligible to apply as an individual institution; hospitals with fewer than 300 beds applied as a consortium of two or more hospitals. Through their Call for Proposal, the two foundations challenged nursing leadership and their executive colleagues to take a risk, shift their paradigms, and use their collective talents and expertise to create a vision and transform their future. More than 1,000 nonprofit, general care hospitals responded. Because of the complexity of institutionwide restructuring, the program was developed in two phases — planning and implementation. The 1,000 hospitals were represented by 608 applications from hospitals or consortia. Of the 608, 80 hospitals or consortia projects were selected for a one-year planning grant of up to $50,000 in October 1989. The 80 projects represented 211 hospitals in 42 states and the District of Columbia. During the planning year, project teams completed a detailed five-year blueprint for restructuring their institutions to promote a patient care delivery system that offered a continuum of care and encompassed characteristics of patient-centeredness, that is, a system designed to meet the needs of the patient and family rather than the needs of the care setting, department, or discipline.

In October 1990, 20 hospitals or consortia were selected for the five-year implementation phase (phase II) of the national program. The 20 projects, representing more than 68 institutions, illustrated the most promising organizational and operational designs for improving patient care. These projects received up to $1 million over a five-year period to complete their demonstration. Eighteen of the original 20 implementation projects continue to demonstrate those designs. (See figure A-1.) The 18 project teams represent more than 65 institutions in 14 states and the District of Columbia. They range in size from small rural institutions to large urban medical centers, both public and private, and include teaching and nonteaching health care systems.

• Program Objectives

SHNP seeks to strengthen patient care and improve relationships of all care providers by addressing the following objectives:

- To foster development of innovative systems to strengthen patient care through collaborative efforts of all patient care providers, including nurses, physicians, other health professionals, and support staff
- To create work environments that optimally use human resources and improve care in a cost-effective and efficient manner
- To establish patterns of service delivery that promote satisfaction among patients, nurses, physicians, and other staff

• Identified Barriers Affecting Optimal Delivery of Patient Care

Early in phase I, participating hospitals and consortia identified a number of internal and external barriers that were affecting optimal care delivery to patients. *Internal barriers* were defined as those existing within the hospital setting, and *external barriers* were defined as interferences outside the hospital, including demographics, regulations, and supply and demand issues. The barriers were reviewed in phase II to determine whether they had changed or no longer existed.

In 1989, 50 percent or more of phase I hospitals and consortia reported the following internal barriers:

- Inadequate nursing resources (85 percent)
- Nursing practice deficits (76 percent)
- Insufficient department support services (76 percent)
- Unmet compensation and benefits needs (63 percent)
- Nursing–physician staff relations (60 percent)
- Lack of nursing management participation in hospitalwide decision making (59 percent)
- Job dissatisfaction (54 percent)

Figure A-1. SHNP Participants

Individual Organizations:

Abbott-Northwestern Hospital, Minneapolis
Beth Israel Hospital, Boston
District of Columbia General Hospital, Washington, DC
Harbor-UCLA Medical Center, Torrance, CA
Hartford Hospital, Hartford, CT
Mercy Hospital and Medical Center, Chicago
MeritCare Hospital, Fargo, ND
Providence Portland Medical Center, Portland, OR
Tallahassee Memorial Regional Medical Center, Tallahassee, FL
University Hospital/Pennsylvania State University, The Milton S. Hershey Medical Center, Hershey, PA
University Hospital/University of Utah Health Science Center, Salt Lake City
Vanderbilt University Hospital and The Vanderbilt Clinic, Nashville

Consortia:

Health BOND, Mankato, MN

    Arlington Municipal Hospital, Arlington, MN
    Immanuel-St. Joseph's Hospital, Mankato, MN
    Mankato State University, Mankato, MN
    Mankato Technical College, Mankato, MN
    Waseca Area Memorial Hospital, Waseca, MN

Mercy Health Services Consortium, Farmington Hills, MI

    Battle Creek Health System, Battle Creek, MI
    Catherine McAuley Health Center, Ann Arbor, MI
    Marian Health Center, Sioux City, IA
    Mercy Health Center, Dubuque, IA
    Mercy Hospital, Cadillac, MI
    Mercy Hospital, Grayling, MI
    Mercy Hospital, Muskegon, MI
    Mercy Hospital, Port Huron, MI
    Mercy Hospitals and Health Services of Detroit, Detroit
    Our Lady of Mercy Hospital, Dyer, IN
    Samaritan Health System, Clinton, IA
    St. Joseph Mercy Hospital, Mason City, IA
    St. Joseph Mercy Hospital, Pontiac, MI
    St. Lawrence Hospital and Healthcare Services, Lansing, MI
    St. Mary's Health Services, Grand Rapids, MI
    Traverse City Osteopathic Hospital, Traverse City, MI

Figure A-1. (Continued)

The Montana Consortium for Excellence in Health Care

Columbus Hospital, Great Falls, MT
Community Memorial Hospital, Sydney, MT
Frances Mahon Deaconess Hospital, Glasglow, MT
Holy Rosary Hospital, Miles City, MT
St. Joseph Hospital, Polson, MT
St. Patrick Hospital, Missoula, MT
St. Vincent Hospital and Health Center, Billings, MT

The Rural Connection: Linking for Healthier Communities

Boise State University, Boise, ID
Holy Rosary Medical Center, Ontario, OR
Idaho Elks Rehabilitation Hospital, Boise, ID
McCall Memorial Hospital, McCall, ID
St. Luke's Regional Medical Center, Boise, ID
Walter Knox Memorial Hospital, Emmett, ID
Wood River Memorial Hospital, Hailey, ID
Wood River Memorial hospital, Sun Valley, ID

University Hospitals of Cleveland, Cleveland and Network Organizations

Geauga Hospital, Chardon, OH
Lakewood Hospital, Lakewood, OH
Lorain Community Hospital, Lorain, OH
Marymount Hospital, Garfield Heights, OH
University MEDNET, Cleveland

Vermont Nursing Initiative

Brattleboro Memorial Hospital, Morrisville, VT
Central Vermont Medical Center, Barre, VT
Copley Hospital, Morrisville, VT
Fanny Allen Hospital, Colchester, VT
Gifford Memorial Hospital, Randolph, VT
Grace Cottage Hospital, Townsend, VT
Medical Center Hospital of Vermont, Burlington, VT
Mt. Ascutney Hospital and Health Center, Windsor, VT
North Country Hospital, Newport, VT
Northeastern Vermont Regional Hospital, St. Johnsbury, VT
Northwestern Medical Center, St. Albans, VT
Porter Medical Center, Middlebury, VT
Rutland Regional Medical Center, Rutland, VT
Southwestern Vermont Medical Center, Bennington, VT
Springfield Hospital, Springfield, VT

By 1991, many of the barriers had shifted from supply and demand issues of the work force to knowledge and skills of the work force—having the right person in the right place to appropriately meet the needs of patients and families. Cost reduction resulting from the reimbursement system and other economic pressures also became a major focus. Job dissatisfaction and tension became an opportunity for change, along with developing relationships beyond hospital walls to include community agencies, educational systems, payers, legislators, and health policymakers. Support service issues, although still important, are resolving as these departments become collaborative members of innovation teams. Nursing involvement in hospital-wide decision making was not mentioned as a significant issue in 1991.[1]

In 1989, the following external barriers were identified:

- Supply–demand imbalance of nurses (74 percent)
- Limitations imposed by reimbursement and other regulatory issues (73 percent)
- Variations in regional/demographic patterns (71 percent)
- Difficulties in recruitment of health care workers (61 percent)

In the 1991 reports, external barriers were identified as being more significant than internal barriers, particularly those related to reimbursement and regulation. Health care reform issues were expressed as the primary concern by everyone—how to shift from traditional reimbursement methods to the anticipated capitated system.[2]

• Themes That Emerged

SHNP institutions brought people together from all levels and many different departments of the organization to develop innovations for improving patient care. Institutional project teams were composed of executive leadership, including the chief executive officer (CEO), the nurse executive, and the chief financial officer (CFO); board of trustee and physician representatives; and multidisciplinary professional care providers and support staff. Although the restructuring efforts for the project teams were diverse, certain consistent themes emerged. These included:

- Delivery systems that offer attributes of patient-centeredness and continuity of care, including case management, collaborative care, integrated clinical practice, care planning, and care-managed, integrated delivery systems of patient care
- Work and role redesign options, including advanced nurse practitioner roles and multicompetent (multiskilled) roles for support staff

- Involvement of information systems, financial systems, human resources, management engineering, environmental services, and other support departments in restructuring processes
- Involvement of executive leadership, physicians, and trustees in restructuring processes
- Linkages between hospitals and other care settings such as home, long-term, preventive, and wellness care resulting in vertical integration of these services
- Linkages with communities; educational institutions including social agencies, high schools, community colleges, and universities; policymakers; and payers

• Interactive Planning: The Fundamental Direction for Change

The SHNP 1989 educational sessions and workshops attended by the grantees were a vital part of their development as change agents and transformational leaders. The CEO, nurse executive, CFO, physician, and trustee representatives and project staff from each grant project attended educational sessions as teams, comprising an audience of more than 500 health care leaders. The stage was set for the first session by Stuart Altman, PhD, from Brandeis University, who established the philosophical foundation for perceiving economic changes that influence the communities, organizations, and individuals personally. Connie Curran, RN, EdD, FAAN, and Marc Roberts, PhD, followed with findings from The Commonwealth Fund paper titled "What to Do about the Nursing Shortage." Russell L. Ackoff, PhD, founder of Interact (The Institute for Interactive Management), set the fundamental direction for change by presenting his interactive planning model. Weaving in both theories and techniques, he mandated an interdisciplinary process through which organizational leaders and employees at all levels of the organization could envision their idealized future, or desired outcome. By using system-age tools rather than machine-age thinking, he showed how the organization needs to involve many disciplines and their leaders in inventing ways to approximate that future.[3] He emphasized the critical role of leadership for seeking alignment of all people for the desired outcome. The 1½-day session was videotaped and a copy sent to each participant in the program's planning and implementation phase, as well as to each of the 528 applicants who did not receive funding.

In an effort to continue the learning process and provide pragmatic, hands-on tools for organizational change, grantee teams attended a two-day workshop held at the University of Pennsylvania's Leonard Davis Institute (LDI) of Health Economics, in Philadelphia. Under the direction of

Sheldon Rovin, DDS, MS, associate director of LDI, and faculty from the Center for Applied Research, the teams learned nominal group technique, an interactive process guaranteed to provide equal time and consideration to all participants regardless of organizational status; stakeholder mapping, a systematic tool used to identify key players; responsibility charting, a method of determining the levels of stakeholder responsibility; project management, techniques for managing all elements of a project, including how to run a meeting, create an agenda, and facilitate meaningful conversation; and the importance of recording minutes and journaling stories for an historical record of their innovations.

The second educational program in April 1991, which built on Ackoff's work, featured Peter M. Senge, PhD, and Charlotte Roberts, principal partners from Innovation Associates in Farmington, Massachusetts. According to Senge and Roberts, creating an ideal future requires building a shared vision with the people involved. They described principles of visionary leadership — for example, people do not have to reach total agreement on what the hospital should do but must agree on its mission and purpose. It is critical to invite people to learn policies and procedures at all levels of the organization so that they can understand the impact of their actions on others and their contribution to the desired outcome. They introduced the language of systems thinking through an assimilated supply–emand game called the Beer Game. They demonstrated the tools of *reinforcing loops* (those that generate growth) and *balancing loops* (those that generate the force of resistance) and applied archetypes such as *fixes that backfire, limits to growth,* and *shifting the burden* to show how problems could be resolved in the work setting of the hospital project team.[4] (These loops, archetypes, and others are presented in a book by Senge and colleagues titled *The Fifth Discipline Fieldbook: Strategies and Tools for Building a Learning Organization.*[5]) As preparation for this program, each institution was given a copy of Senge's book *The Fifth Discipline: The Art and Practice of Learning Organizations.* This session also was videotaped and copies given to the planning and implementation hospitals and consortia. Because this session was designed for phase II of the program, only the implementation institutions attended, comprising an audience of more than 200 health care leaders.

The third educational session teamed Donald N. Lombardi, PhD, the principal partner of CHR/Intervista, Inc., of Hackettstown, New Jersey, and Thomas N. Gilmore, PhD, vice-president, Center for Applied Research, in Philadelphia. Phase II grant projects were again represented by CEOs, nurse executives, medical staff representatives, trustee representatives, and project staff, along with CFOs and leaders of other departments such as information systems, human resources, education and research, and management engineering.

Lombardi began this session with his work in value-driven management. According to Lombardi, value-driven management is the basis of *progressive management,* a term he uses to describe the management activities and strategies of an effective health care manager at any level of an organization.[6] He focused on management of human resources, delineating specific situations that confront managers. The audience learned about alternatives for achieving higher levels of performance by using value-driven strategies such as customer community strategies and organizational business strategies.

Building on Lombardi's work, Gilmore provided grantee teams an opportunity to think about dilemmas of institutionalizing innovations. Through interactive dialogue within grantee teams, he asked teams to think about tension that exists between parallel (ad hoc) structures developed to generate new ideas and the ongoing operational structures used to carry out business as usual. He emphasized that innovation requires freedom from existing organizational structures. Ideas coming from many sources — health care consumers, community leaders, care providers, and new organizational leaders and staff — need structure in which to germinate and evolve. Ad hoc structures often are put in place to develop those new ideas, plan for implementation, set targets, and monitor performance. These ad hoc structures can bring drawbacks and dangers, especially if the desired end is a new organizational culture. The resulting tension requires energy, attention, and commitment from key leadership to enable emergence of an enduring change.[7,8]

Each SHNP organization developed its own educational program to share the learnings from the national education programs and to continue learning as each pursued its projects. External consultants often were utilized to facilitate, mentor, and coach these programs. Each organization's goal was to use the consultant to teach its leaders how to carry on their own programs and to do their work. Organizations that did not initiate an institutionwide developmental program early did so later and found that their vision was not institutionalized until all levels of managers and staff had experienced the process.

• Factors for Success

The following successful factors were consistently demonstrated by individual hospitals and consortia:

- The hospital or consortium has a substantive, shared vision known by people at all levels of the organization.
- The organization's executive management, board of trustees, and key physicians are committed and actively involved in the change process.
- The change process is interactive, involving individuals from many different levels and departments within and outside the organization.
- The change process is based on principles of interactive processes, systems thinking, learning organization, and quality improvement.

- The patient care delivery system innovations are patient centered across the continuum of care.
- Decision making is pushed to the level of the organization closest to the patient and, when appropriate, involves the patient and his or her family.
- The hospital/health care system has undergone a shift in organizational culture and is open to continuous learning, improving, and adapting.

• Lessons Learned from the Project Teams

Learning is an essential component of the national program. Lessons include:

- The process used to achieve the desired outcomes should become the template or model for future solutions. (Each health care setting has its own internal and external factors to consider. Although processes for innovation will be similar, the desired outcome must fit each unique environment.)
- Significant early educational time should be designed for people at all levels of the organization, including managers and care providers.
- Physicians should be involved early on in the change process. Change is crucial to them and significantly affects their practices.
- Key departments such as information systems, human resources, financial systems, environmental engineering, and management engineering should be involved in planning and implementation of restructuring projects.
- A common language should be established and institutionalized.
- Open communication, dialogue, relationship building, consensus decision making, systems thinking, and interactive processes should be recognized as essential to a change process.
- Individual accountability should shift to team accountability, creating a collective "we" for achieving the desired outcome.
- A mechanism should be established to clarify professional and support staff roles and to design new roles based on the work of patient care.
- Dissatisfaction or tension should be expected and encouraged; dissatisfaction can bring questions and new ideas if open communication is encouraged.
- The competencies of everyone involved should be understood, recognizing the unique talents that each person brings to the change process as well as each individual's accountability for the desired outcome.
- Trustee-approved restructuring should be integrated as part of the organizational strategic plan and trustee representatives should be actively involved.
- Linkages should be developed emphasizing the continuum of care with communities, educational institutions at all levels, and payers and policy-makers.

- Measurements should be developed to demonstrate the cost impact of institutionwide restructuring and gains for the patient, employee, and organization.

• Evaluation Design for an Organization Experiencing Change

SHNP institutions selected their particular change project based on perceived needs and culture, the population they serve, and their internal diversity. Because projects are different, critical indicators demonstrating effectiveness differ among institutions. SHNP recommended that the evaluation design fit the individual institution and be responsive to changes as they occur throughout the life of the project and in the environment. The design should produce useful knowledge derived from real-world experiences and allow for a better understanding of restructuring efforts. The design that seemed most acceptable to the project teams is based on principles of action learning or action research as well as elements of experimental design. Many institutions integrated evaluation of their project with continuous quality improvement efforts. Project teams found that experimental design alone is inadequate, because it requires too many controls and does not readily support a fluid, dynamic process. Action research uses case studies, interviews, surveys, meeting minutes, journals, anecdotal stories, and operational management reports as its data sources. Often there are no standards with which to compare the work. However, through constant and consistent data collection, internal trends with which to compare their work over time are established.

• Expansion of Relationships

The SHNP hospitals and consortia are connecting with elementary schools, high schools, community colleges, and universities to establish relationships and jointly plan preparation of the health care worker for the future. They are communicating these educational needs to local and national policymakers and legislators. Some institutions invited legislators and licensing officials to participate as members of planning and implementation committees that address work force needs.

Institutions are working directly with payers in local communities and negotiating reimbursement for outpatient services not covered previously. These efforts are resulting in reduced hospital stays and lower overall cost for service, as well as placing the patient in more comfortable care environments, including the home.

Although they initially focused on hospital care, all projects broadened the scope of work to include care settings outside the hospital, as well as social service agencies. There is commitment to integrate care across all settings, including home, rehabilitative, long-term, wellness, and preventive care. This scope has refocused projects from hospital-based to community-based services with intent to support development of models for a healthier community.

References

1. National Program Office. *Strengthening Hospital Nursing: A Program to Improve Patient Care, Gaining Momentum: A Progress Report.* St. Petersburg, FL: The Robert Wood Johnson Foundation and The Pew Charitable Trusts, 1992.

2. National Program Office. *Strengthening Hospital Nursing: A Program to Improve Patient Care National Meeting Brochure and Resource Materials.* St. Petersburg, FL: The Robert Wood Johnson Foundation and The Pew Charitable Trusts, Fall 1994.

3. Ackoff, R. L. *Creating the Corporate Future.* New York City: John Wiley and Sons, 1981.

4. Senge, P. M. *The Fifth Discipline: The Art and Practice of the Learning Organization.* New York City: Doubleday, 1990.

5. Senge, P. M., Roberts, C., Ross, R. B., Smith, B. J., and Kleiner, A. *The Fifth Discipline Fieldbook: Strategies and Tools for Building a Learning Organization.* New York City: Doubleday, 1994.

6. Lombardi, D. *Progressive Health Care Management Strategies.* Chicago: American Hospital Publishing, 1992.

7. Gilmore, T. N. Dilemmas of institutionalizing transformations. SHNP education program, Orlando, FL, Sept. 1993.

8. Gilmore, T. N., and Krantz, J. Innovations in the public sector: dilemmas in the use of ad hoc process. *Journal of Policy Analysis and Management* 10(3):455–68, Summer 1991.

Appendix B

Suggested Resources

This appendix of suggested resources is divided into two sections. The first section lists books and articles of general interest; the second section lists books and other media that focus more specifically on leadership development.

• General Interest

Ackoff, R. L. *Creating the Corporate Future.* New York City: John Wiley and Sons, 1981.

Aiken, L., and Fagin, C. *Charting Nursing's Agenda for the 1990s.* Philadelphia: J. P. Lippincott Co., 1992.

American Organization of Nurse Executives. *Nursing Leadership: Preparing for the 21st Century.* Chicago: American Hospital Publishing, 1993.

Bolman, L. G., and Deal, T. E. Merger meltdown. *Healthcare Forum Journal* 37(6):30–36, Nov.–Dec. 1994.

Bowers, M. R., Swan, J. E., and Koehler, W. F. What attributes determine quality and satisfaction with health care delivery. *Healthcare Management Review* 19(4):49–55, Fall 1994.

Bridging the Leadership Gap in Healthcare. Executive Summary of a National Study Conducted by the Leadership Center of the Healthcare Forum. San Francisco: The Healthcare Forum, 1992.

Calvert, G. *Hire Wire Management: Risk-Taking for Leaders, Innovators, and Trailblazers.* San Francisco: Jossey-Bass, 1993.

Charns, M. P., and Smith Tewksbury, L. J. *Collaborative Management in Health Care: Implementing the Integrative Organization.* San Francisco: Jossey-Bass, 1993.

Cohen, E. L., and Cesta, T. G. *Nursing Case Management: From Concept to Evaluation.* St. Louis: Mosby, 1993.

Coile, R. C. The five stages of managed care: organizing for capitation and health reform. *Hospital Strategy,* 6(11):1–8, Sept. 1994.

Coile, R. C. The sixth stage of managed care: 10 models for the post reform era. *Hospital Strategy Report* 7(1):1–8, Nov. 1994.

Companies discover downside to downsizing. *St. Petersburg Times,* July 6, 1994, section E.

Connor, R. D. Bouncing back: resilience as the essential component that transforms the reality of organizational change into a manageable process. *SKY* 23(9):30–34, Sept. 1994.

Covey, S. R. *The 7 Habits of Highly Effective People: Powerful Lessons in Personal Change.* New York City: Simon and Schuster, 1990.

de Bono, E. *Lateral Thinking: Creativity Step by Step.* New York City: Harper and Row, 1970.

Drucker, P. F. *The Five Most Important Questions You Will Ever Ask about Your Nonprofit Organization.* San Francisco: Jossey-Bass, 1993.

Drucker, P. F. *Managing for the Future: The 1990s and Beyond.* New York City: Truman Tally Books/Dutton, 1992.

Dumaine, B. Mr. learning organization. *Fortune* 130(8):147–57, Oct. 17, 1994.

Eisler, R. *The Chalice and the Blade: Our History, Our Future.* San Francisco, Harper and Row, 1988.

Flarey, D. L. *Redesigning Nursing Care Delivery.* Philadelphia: J. B. Lippincott Co., 1994.

Freudenheim, M. Health industry is changing itself ahead of reform. *The New York Times,* June 27, 1994, section A.1, column 4.

Gilmore, T. N. Dilemmas of institutionalizing transformations. SHNP education program, Orlando, FL, Sept. 1993.

Gilmore, T. N., and Krantz, J. Innovations in the public sector: dilemmas in the use of ad hoc process. *Journal of Policy Analysis and Management* 10(3):455–68, Summer 1991.

Goldberg, N. *Long Quiet Highway: Waking Up in America.* New York City: Bantam Books, 1993.

Hamel, G., and Prahalad, C. K. Seeing the future first. *Fortune* 130(5):64–70, Sept. 5, 1994.

The Health Care Forum Leadership Center's Healthier Communities Partnership. *Healthier Communities Action Kit: A Guide for Leaders Embracing Change.* Module 1. San Francisco: The Healthcare Forum, 1993.

Ill, P. The passion to lead: transforming accomplishment into achievement. *Administrative Radiology Journal* 13(7):25–28, July 1994.

Infusino, D. The reluctant guru. *American Way* 27(12):70–112, June 15, 1994.

Inguagiato, R. *Organizational Theory: Fundamentals of Medical Management.* Tampa: American College of Physician Executives, 1993.

Jacks, G., and Hunt, C. T. *Patient-Centered Care: Everyone's Business.* Washington, DC: District of Columbia General Hospital, 1994.

Kanter, M. R. *The Change Masters: Innovation and Entrepreneurship in the American Corporation.* New York City: Simon and Schuster, 1983.

Kanter, M. R. Collaborative advantages: the art of alliances. *Harvard Business Review* 72(4):96–108, July–Aug. 1994.

Kohles, M. K., and Donaho, B. A. Twenty grantees seek transformation: from discipline-driven compartmentalized entities to patient-driven, unified care systems. *Strategies for Health Care Excellence* 5(11):1–12, Nov. 1992.

Leebov, W., and Scott, G. *Health Care Managers in Transition: Shifting Roles and Changing Organizations.* San Francisco: Jossey-Bass, 1990.

Marszalek-Gaucher, E., and Coffey, R. *Transforming Healthcare Organizations: How to Achieve and Sustain Organizational Excellence.* San Francisco: Jossey-Bass, 1990.

Moore, N., and Komras, H. *Patient-Focused Healing: Integrating Caring and Curing in Health Care.* San Francisco: Jossey-Bass, 1993.

Morgan, G. *Imaginization: The Art of Creative Management*. Newbury Park, CA: Sage Publications, 1993.

Morgan, G. *Personal Communication*. Newbury Park, CA: Sage Publications, 1995.

National Program Office. *Strengthening Hospital Nursing: A Program to Improve Patient Care, Gaining Momentum: A Progress Report*. St. Petersburg, FL: The Robert Wood Johnson Foundation and The Pew Charitable Trusts, 1992.

National Program Office. *Strengthening Hospital Nursing: A Program to Improve Patient Care National Meeting Brochure and Meeting Resource Notebook*. St. Petersburg, FL: The Robert Wood Johnson Foundation and The Pew Charitable Trusts, Fall 1994.

Patton, M. Q. *Practical Evaluation*. Newbury Park, CA: Sage Publications, 1982.

Porter-O'Grady, T. *Creative Nursing Administration: Participative Management into the 21st Century*. Rockville, MD: Aspen Publishers, 1986.

Rothstein, L. R. The empowerment effort that came undone. *Harvard Business Review* 73(1):20–31, Jan.–Feb. 1995.

Rovin, S., and Ginsberg, L. *Managing Hospitals: Lessons from The Johnson & Johnson-Wharton Fellows Program in Management for Nurses*. San Francisco: Jossey-Bass, 1991.

Schon, D. *Educating the Reflective Practitioner*. San Francisco: Jossey-Bass, 1987.

Sherman, S. Leaders learn to heed the voice within. *Fortune,* pp. 92–100, Aug. 22, 1994.

Shortell, S., Gillies, R. B., Anderson, D. A., Mitchell, J. D., and Morgan, K. L. Creating organized delivery systems: the barriers and facilitators. *Hospital & Health Services Administration* 38(4):447–66, Winter 1993.

Shortell, S. M., Morrison, E. M., and Friedman, B. *Strategic Choices for America's Hospitals: Managing Change in Turbulent Times*. San Francisco: Jossey-Bass, 1992.

Starr, P. *The Social Transformation of American Medicine: The Rise of a Sovereign Profession and the Making of a Vast Industry*. New York City: Basic Books, 1982.

Stein, M., and Hollwitz, J. *Psyche at Work: Workplace Applications of Jungian Analytical Psychology.* Wilmette, IL: Chiron Publications, 1992.

Stevens, R. *In Sickness and in Wealth: American Hospitals in the Twentieth Century.* San Francisco: Basic Books, 1989.

Stewart, T. A. How to lead a revolution. *Fortune* 130(11):48–61, Nov. 28, 1994.

Storm, H. *Lightningbolt.* New York City: Ballantine Books, 1994.

Strengthening 1(1), Spring 1992.

Umbdenstock, R. J., and Hageman, W. M. *Critical Readings for Hospital Trustees.* Chicago: American Hospital Publishing, 1991.

Waterman, R. H., Waterman, J. A., and Collard, B. Toward a career-resilient workforce. *Harvard Business Review* 72(4):87–95, July–Aug. 1994.

Weisbord, M. *Discovering Common Ground.* San Francisco: Berrett-Koehler, 1992.

Whiteside, J. *The Phoenix Agenda.* Essex Junction, VT: Oliver Wright Publications, 1993.

Whyte, D. *The Heart Aroused: Poetry and the Preservation of the Soul in Corporate America.* New York City: Doubleday, 1994.

Yetton, P. W., Johnston, K. D., and Craig, J. F. Computer-aided architects: a case study of IT and strategic change. *Sloan Management Review* 35(4):57–65, Summer 1994.

• Leadership Development

When an individual has no clear leadership development goals, it is easy to become disappointed, give up, or vacillate in his or her resolve to grow. To have direction, it is necessary to understand oneself. This enhances self-esteem, strengthens self-confidence, decreases feelings of self-doubt, and supports growth toward self-mastery. Self-mastery is key to developing effective relationships; and because successful leaders rely on effective and appropriate relationships, self-mastery is fundamental to all developmental processes for transformational leadership. The character traits essential for effective interpersonal relationships are integrity, honesty, trustworthiness, dignity, and maturity. As these traits are valued and modeled by transformational leaders, others in the organization will respect their worth and adopt similar behaviors in their own interactions.

How are self-mastery and effective leadership traits learned? The learning process involves a number of steps:

1. Having the desire to learn and change behaviors and attitudes, and knowing that change is possible
2. Recognizing that there is no one way to learn and that learning is the synthesis of both formal educational and informal life experiences to produce new insights
3. Understanding that mistakes, even failures, are part of learning and building self-confidence
4. Letting go of perfection and accepting that "good enough" allows for improvement and achievement of potential
5. Allowing time to nourish the soul and spiritual part of one's self

Processes, opportunities, and tools for developing self-mastery and effective leadership traits are multiple and will constantly evolve as more is learned about self-understanding and self-knowledge.

Rather than list tools, processes, and opportunities for leadership development, this appendix suggests several key sources and resources that are available for finding out about such information. Exciting new materials are published frequently, and regular trips to local and/or college bookstores will enhance familiarity with new selections in fields such as business, anthropology, philosophy, psychology, and other special studies. Additionally, *The York Times* best-seller list and other news media can be helpful in determining what materials others are reading.

Books

Continuous Quality Improvement, Outcomes Management, Reengineering, Restructuring, and Work and Role Redesign

Coan, T. Reengineering the organization: an approach for discontinuous change. *Quality Management in Health Care* 2(3):15–26, Spring 1994.

Delbecq, A. L., Van de Ven, A. H., and Gustafson, D. H. *Group Techniques and Program Planning: A Guide to Nominal Group Technique and Delphi Process.* Glenview, IL: Scott Foresman, 1975.

Hammer, M., and Champy, J. *Reengineering the Corporation: A Manifesto for Business Revolution.* New York City: HarperCollins, 1993.

Hanson, R. B., and Sayers, B. *Work and Role Redesign: Tools and Techniques for the Health Care Setting.* Chicago: American Hospital Publishing, 1995.

Leebov, W., and Ersoz, C. J. *The Health Care Manager's Guide to Continuous Quality Improvement.* Chicago: American Hospital Publishing, 1991.

Melum, M. M., and Sinioris, M. K. *Total Quality Management: The Health Care Pioneers.* Chicago: American Hospital Publishing, 1992.

Scholtes, P. R. *The Team Handbook.* Madison, WI: Joiner Associates, 1992.

Spath, P. L., editor. *Clinical Paths: Tools for Outcomes Management.* Chicago: American Hospital Publishing, 1994.

Conversation and Dialogue

Bohm, D. *On Dialogue.* Ojai, CA: David Bohm Seminars, 1990.

Isaacs, W. N. *Taking Flight: Dialogue, Collective Thinking, and Organizational Learning. Dia•Logos.* Cambridge, MA: Organizational Learning Center at Massachusetts Institute of Technology, 1994.

Schein, E. H. *On Dialogue: Culture and Organizational Learning. Dia•Logos.* Cambridge, MA: Institute for Generative Learning and Collaborative Social Change, 1994, pp. 46–51.

Interactive Planning and Management, Learning Organization, Organizational Development, Systems Thinking, and Value Management

Ackoff, R. L., Finnel, E. V., and Gharajedaghi, J. *A Guide to Controlling Your Corporation's Future.* New York City: John Wiley and Sons, 1984.

Cummings, T. G., and Worley, C. G. *Organization Development and Change.* 5th ed. St. Paul: West Publishing Co., 1993.

Gibson, J. L., Ivancevich, J. M., and Donnelly, Jr., J. H. Organizations, Behavior, Structure, Process. 8th ed. Burr Ridge, IL: Richard D. Irwin, Inc., 1994.

Lombardi, D. *Progressive Management Health Care Strategies.* Chicago: American Hospital Publishing, 1992.

Ray, M., and Rinzler, A., editors. *The New Paradigm in Business.* New York City: Jeremy P. Tarcher/Perigee Books, 1993.

Senge, P. M., Roberts, C., Ross, R. B., Smith, B. J., and Kleiner, A. *The Fifth Discipline Fieldbook: Strategies and Tools for Building a Learning Organization.* New York City: Doubleday, 1994.

Senge, P. M. *The Fifth Discipline: The Art and Practice of the Learning Organization.* New York City: Doubleday, 1990.

Principle-Centered and Visionary Leadership

Bennis, W. *An Invented Life: Reflections on Leadership and Change.* Reading, MA: Addison-Wesley Publishing Co., 1993.

Capra, F. *The Turning Point: Science, Society, and the Rising Culture.* New York City: Bantam Books, 1982.

Covey, S. R. *Principle-Centered Leadership.* New York City: Simon & Schuster, 1992.

Kaiser, L. R. *Lifework Planning.* Brighton, CO: Brighton Books, Nov. 1989, pp. 1–7.

Kaiser, L. R. The visionary manager. In: T. C. Wilson, editor. *Emerging Issues in Health Care 1988.* Estes Park, CO: Estes Park Institute, 1988.

Owen, H. *Leadership Is.* Potomac, MD: Abbott Publishing, 1990.

Wheatley, M. J. *Leadership and the New Science: Learning about Organization from an Orderly Universe.* San Francisco: Berrett-Koehler, 1992.

Project Management and Management Development

Graham, R. J. *Project Management As If People Mattered.* Bala Cynwyd, PA: Primavera Press, 1989.

Schmeling, W. M. *Management/Staff Development.* Chicago: American Hospital Publishing, 1995.

Stetler, C. B., and Charns, M. P. *Collaboration in Health Care: Hartford Hospital's Experience in Changing Management and Practice.* Chicago: American Hospital Publishing, 1995.

Soul Work

Cousineau, P., editor. *Soul: An Archaeology.* San Francisco: Harpers, 1994.

Moore, T. *Care of the Soul.* New York City: HarperCollins, 1992.

Moore, T. *Soulmates: Honoring the Mysteries of Lvoe and Relationship.* New York City: HarperCollins, 1994.

Peck, M. S. *A World Waiting to Be Born: Civility Rediscovered.* New York City: Bantam Books, 1993.

Tinder, G. *Against Fate: An Essay on Personal Dignity.* Notre Dame, IN: University of Notre Dame Press, 1981.

Wallis, J. *The Soul of Politics.* Maryknoll, NY: The New Press and Orbis Books, 1994.

Health Care Journals

Administrative Radiology Journal, Case Management Review, Healthcare Forum, Hospitals and Health Care Systems, Hospitals & Health Services Administration, Hospital Strategy Report, Journal of Nursing Administration, Journal of Quality Assurance, Modern Health Care, Quality Management Review, and other specialty health care journals

Newspapers and Magazines

New York Times, The Wall Street Journal and local community newspapers; *Newsweek, Times, U. S. News and World Report,* and other magazines

Business News and Journals

Business Week, Forbes Magazine, Fortune, Harvard Business Review, Sloan Management Review and others

Alternative Journals

Harper's Magazine, New Age Journal, North America Review, The Nation, The Progressive, Public Culture, Sierra, Sojourners, Utne Reader, airline magazines, and others

Electronic Networks

- CompuServe™, CONNECT™, Internet, and HandsNet™ are examples of networks offering a variety of services.
- MCI Mail and AT&T Mail specialize in mail services.
- DIALOG and NEXIS provide on-line data bases for retrieval of specific information such as daily health news, specialized publications, abstracts, and statistics on almost any subject.

Appendix C

Glossary

Definitions for the following terms have been formulated combining author and contributor wording and the language found in current organizational development literature.

"Ah ha" experience: A watershed or breakthrough experience; the moment when one's vision suddenly expands from a narrow focus to a broader view. It is the point at which an individual or group has new insight into a situation.

Archetype: An energy pattern or most basic structure. The essence for an archetype is within the person, organization, and community. It is the unique person you are designed to be or the uniqueness of the organization as a composite of the people who provide or receive service.

Cocreation: A process in which people work together for the purpose of producing a common desired outcome. It is based on systems thinking and interactive principles and is synergistic, meaning that the whole is greater than the sum of its parts. It promotes the use of imagination, dreams, innovations, and visions, and moves a group (often an interdisciplinary team) from a cooperative relationship to one of collaboration and interdependence. Cocreation usually starts as a personal vision that becomes a group's shared vision. It is a process for creating "teamness." Intellectual, emotional, societal, and spiritual dimensions of individuals and the team are part of the cocreation process; and trust, mutual respect, and dialogue are essential elements.

Consensus building: A rational means of decision making in which individuals seek to limit options and focus on those acceptable to the entire group or team. Consensus building produces a result that "everyone can live with," but does not necessarily alter the fundamental differences that led people to disagree in the first place.

Continuum (continuity) of care: A seamless flow of patient care services across a variety of care settings such as home, long-term, preventive, maintenance, and wellness. Terms such as *longitudinal integration* or *vertical integration* also refer to continuums of care that may include multiple institutions or systems and their communities. Continuity of care that is patient centered means that care across settings is patient needs responsive. The continuum of care approach encourages constancy of relationships among patient, family, and care providers which may be maintained through an interconnected communication system or a single, constant care provider such as a nurse or other professional (for example, a case manager).

Destiny: Similar to *soul,* which may be understood as the essential self, transcendent and sacred. A destiny is simultaneously personal and communal. Destiny is a direction coming from beyond the individual or organizational environment. The counterconcept of destiny is fate, which is broadly conceived as all that threatens human dignity. To speak of personal or organizational destiny is to speak of that which must somehow come to fruition in the struggle against fate. In health care, the authors believe that patient-centered care restores human dignity in this context.

Dialogue: The flow of meaning that among us and between us leads to new understanding; from the Greek word *dialogos,* in which *logos* translates as "the meaning of the word" and *dia* means" through." Dialogue seeks to have people learn how to think together. Dialogue is more than consensus in that participants gain insights into the fundamental patterns that lead to differences as they participate in creation of shared new meaning.

Facilitator role: An influencing role in which the facilitator is neither authoritarian nor abdicator, but encourages desired outcomes.

Interactive planning and management process: A process that identifies opportunities for desired operational and clinical improvements. *Current reality* (the way it is presently) and *desired future* (what is wanted) are defined and the differences show opportunities for improvement. Analysis considers both the strengths and limitations of a situation, practice, or issue. Obstacles that interfere with or prevent the desired outcome from being realized are defined along with the means and resources needed to develop and implement the appropriate intervention to prioritize which interventions (inventions) will be pursued. Implementation can be a pilot demonstration before institutionalization. Assessment evaluates the appropriateness and efficacy of the intervention leading to revision new potentials. Time is taken to celebrate the success of the effort. The concepts and principles of continuous quality improvement, interactive processes, learning organizations, strategic thinking, systems thinking, and other management tools and strategies often are used during the management process. Interactive planning and management is based on the work of Russell L. Ackoff of Interact, Inc., with applications by Alan M. Barstow of Barstow and Associates.

Leadership: Creating opportunities to liberate people and organizations to realize their full potentials. Leadership encourages action by people and organizations to achieve positive outcomes of what is desired and helps them foster positive attitudes and behaviors in themselves and others. Leadership honors the soul of persons and experiences by being attentive to preserving human dignity. It involves having a passion for what one believes and does to fulfill personal and institutional destiny. Leadership grows appropriate structure by honoring the openness of insights and spirit and yet maintaining boundaries and encouraging new forms.

Mission: A clear, definable, and motivational point of focus for an organization clarifying its purpose or destiny. Mission guides the organization to select appropriate opportunities toward an achievable desired outcome.

Opportunity: A desired outcome that preserves human dignity and brings enhancement and added value to patients and their families, care providers and other individuals, the organization, and the community.

Organizational development: A process using behavioral science knowledge and practices to help organizations achieve greater effectiveness, including desired outcomes for patients and their families, improved quality of work life for stakeholders, and improved health status for the community and society as a whole. It is a practice oriented toward major change within the total system considering the context of the larger environment that influences the organization.

Patient-centeredness: A philosophy of care referring to a care delivery system designed to meet the needs of the patient and family, rather than the needs of a care setting, department, or discipline involved in providing a service. It is a patient needs–responsive approach to health care services.

Prospector: A leader or an organization able to perceive what needs to change and quickly effect that change. Prospectors move beyond being proactive by perceiving, adapting, and responding in a very short time frame using strategic thinking and behaviors, often assuming more risk than those who are proactive. They are attentive to the future while learning from the past.

Relationship: A connection between people, organizations, communities, and beyond. The visioning and implementation of new opportunities may influence the formation of new, or strengthen existing, relationships resulting in individuals feeling better about themselves (intrapersonal), individuals relating differently to others (interpersonal), or organizational units and departments relating differently to each other (intraorganizational). New or improved relationships between health care institutions (interorganizational) or between institutions and segments of the community (intrasocietal) may develop.

Soul: The essence of an individual, organization, or community, closely aligned with the concept of destiny. Attention to soul improves quality of life. Soul manifests itself through a language of image and symbols, and thrives under conditions of intimacy, attachment, and involvement. Leaders concerned about individual and organizational soul appreciate fantasy, imagination, and creativity, and view relationships as the place where soul works out its destiny.

Stakeholder: A person or group either inside and outside the organization who has the potential to be affected by change.

Strategic thinking: A creative, imaginative, and intuitive way of thinking involving synthesis of informal and formal learning to produce new insights. It encourages dialogue, collaboration, and continued learning.

Systems thinking: Methods, tools, and principles for understanding the interrelatedness of forces, patterns, functions, and elements in an environment. Systems thinking allows people to see internal and external forces in an environment as a part of a common process. A way of thinking and behaving differently from traditional mechanistic approaches, it believes that everything is interrelated and connected. Systems thinking can move a team sharing a common goal from pragmatic and analytical focus to mystical and spiritual dimensions.

Teamness: The collective "we," meaning the process of connecting relationships between people who come together to build a shared vision and develop and implement actions or strategies toward a desired outcome. Teamness is based on trust and mutual respect for the talents and competencies each person brings to the process. A group or team that has achieved teamness has matured to collaborative and interdependent relationships. Members of such a team often describe a feeling of "making a difference," even though they may not always define what that difference is.

The value framework process: Based on the management science of multiattribute utility decision analysis, it relies on the subjective judgment aspect of analysis and provides structure to ask the right questions of people at all levels of the organization in order to define organizational values and objectives in an unambiguous, usable manner. The process gives people the opportunity to identify the basic values of the organization, understand how these values interrelate, and recognize the trade-offs between conflicting values. The process allows people to know how their performance affects the performance of the system to maximize those values and provides the structure to measure performance in relation to those values.

Transformation: To change the function, form, or nature of something; to become liberated, putting aside old existence and creating openness for new expressions to emerge. Transformation is not without pain and disappointment.

Transformational leader: One who freely generates and exchanges ideas, visions, and learnings, and provides opportunities for others to excel and realize their potential. The transformational leader willingly lets go of old patterns and assumptions, and invites new thinking and behaving. Risk taking, inquiry, exploration, and innovation are encouraged; mistakes are considered opportunities for learning. A transformational leader has an active imagination, and places value on the imagination of others.

Value: Greater quality yields increased value, and lower cost represents better value.

Values: Behaviors, characteristics, standards, and viewpoints that are meaningful to a person or an organization; guidelines and beliefs that determine a personal view of the world. Values are rational and irrational judgments and ideals guiding organizational purpose. They give direction to alternatives or opportunities that are considered for an outcome. Often internalized and emotionally laden, they can become so identified with feelings, thinking, attitudes, and behaving that it is not always obvious that they exist. Values tell what a person or organization stands for.

Vision: An intuitive view and knowledge of what people and organizations should be and do, giving direction and meaning; a forceful motivator for change. A visioning process helps define the mission of an organization and clarifies desired outcomes and opportunities to be achieved, although the ideal vision is never fully achieved.

Additional Books of Interest

Breakthrough Leadership: Achieving Organizational Alignment through Hoshin Planning
by Mara Minerva Melum and Casey Collett
Copublished by GOAL/QPC

This book introduces you to a strategy that can help you achieve lasting, organizationwide improvements. With hoshin planning, the full power of people throughout the organization is focused on achieving the organization's most important priorities. Employees at every level understand how they will contribute to those priorities. Progress through such collaboration is often made in quantum leaps.

Catalog no. E99-169108 (must be included when ordering)
1995. 300 pages, 125 figures, 3 appendixes, glossary, bibliography, index.
$69.00 (AHA members, $55.00)

Work and Role Redesign: Tools and Techniques for the Health Care Setting
by Ruth Bredlie Hanson, MS, RN, and Betty Sayers, MS

It's a struggle to redesign work roles and responsibilities to improve efficiency and effectiveness. This book helps ease that struggle by showing you how to tap into and take advantage of an underutilized resource — the vast knowledge and experience of your employees. By using the ideas in this book, you'll be able to unleash the creative problem-solving abilities of the people closest to the customer.

Catalog no. E99-067102 (must be included when ordering)
1995. 216 pages, 39 figures, 13 tables, 2 appendixes.
$49.00 (AHA members, $39.00)

To order, call TOLL FREE
1-800-AHA-2626